D1064551

NEURO-MUSCULAR TECHNIQUE

An authoritative textbook dealing with soft tissue manipulation—a
diagnostic and therapeutic method which restores the structural,
functional and postural integrity of the body, removing pain,
muscular tension, stress and restrictions to health.

By the same author
ABOUT LAETRILE
THE ACUPUNCTURE TREATMENT OF PAIN
AND END TO CANCER?
INSTANT PAIN CONTROL
OSTEOPATHY
RELAXATION AND MEDITATION TECHNIQUES

NEURO-MUSCULAR TECHNIQUE

A Practitioner's Guide to Soft Tissue Manipulation

by
LEON CHAITOW N.D., D.O., M.B.N.O.A.
Illustrated by Bevil Roberts

THORSONS PUBLISHERS LIMITED
Wellingborough, Northamptonshire

THORSONS PUBLISHERS INC.
New York

First published 1980
Second Impression 1983

British Library Cataloguing in Publication Data

Chaitow, Leon
  Neuro-muscular technique.
  1. Manipulation (Therapeutics)
  I. Title
  615'.822   RM701
  ISBN 0-7225-0586-8

Printed and bound in Great Britain

CONTENTS

To my wife, Alkmini and our
daughter, Sasha.

ACKNOWLEDGEMENTS

My grateful thanks go to Dr Boris Chaitow for the notes, photographs and guidance which greatly aided me in the preparation of the chapter on abdominal technique in particular and the whole book in general. I also wish to express my thanks to Peter Lief D.O. for his permission to quote from his written and spoken comments on his and his late father's contribution to manipulative therapy. My thanks go, too, to Brian Youngs B.Sc., D.O. for his generous permission to quote from his authoritative articles on the theoretical and practical aspects of Neuro-muscular Technique. Also, my special thanks to Terry G. Moule N.D., D.O. for his contribution to Chapter 9 'NMT in Clinical Use'.

I acknowledge with gratitude Michael M. Patterson Ph.D., Associate Professor of Osteopathic Medicine at The College of Osteopathic Medicine, Ohio University, for his assistance in giving permission to quote from his writings. My thanks, also, to Churchill Livingstone for permission to quote from the book *Connective Tissue Massage* by Maria Ebner (a book now sadly out of print).

Thanks are also due to the Rolf Institute's Executive Director, Richard Stenstadvold, for permission to quote from the writings of the late founder of the Institute, Ida Rolf; to The Japan Publishing Company for their permission to quote from *Tsubo—Vital Points for Oriental Therapy* by Katsusuke Serizawa M.D.; to Randolph Stone D.C. for the quotations from his work on Polarity Therapy—there is a lot of common ground between his methods and those of Stanley Lief; and to Williams & Wilkins Co. for muscle tests quoted from *Posture and Pain* by Kendall, Kendall and Boynton.

My sincere thanks go to all the writers, medical, osteopathic, chiropractic and others, whose work I have alluded to or quoted from; and especially Bevil Roberts for his dedicated work in illustrating this book.

On a more personal level I wish to thank my father, Max Chaitow, for providing the information regarding the early family history of his cousin Stanley Lief; and to thank most sincerely my wife, Alkmini, without whose patient help this book would not have been written.

Finally, and most importantly, I wish to express my thanks and deep respect to the memory of that giant among men, the late Stanley Lief. His work goes on, and the spread of the knowledge of Neuro-muscular Technique serves to underline yet further his contribution to natural healing. I hope I have done him justice.

INTRODUCTION

The role of the soft tissue of the body in terms of health and dysfunction deserves re-emphasis, as does the relationship of the muscle, fascia and connective tissue in general to the overall economy of the body and to its ability to function efficiently. The ways in which dysfunction in the soft tissue mirrors deeper pathology of both mind and body, and the ways in which it influences such pathology, directly or reflexly, are profoundly important.

A factor common to the various reflex systems (such as acupuncture points, Chapman's neurolymphatic reflexes, myofascial trigger points etc.) seems to be their siting in fascial tissue. The stresses and strains produced in this ubiquitous tissue produce definite patterns, many of which are related to lines of postural stress, which are fairly uniform in man. Andrew Taylor Still, the founder of osteopathic medicine, was clearly prophetic when he stated that the fascia is the place to look for the cause of disease, and the place to begin the action of remedies. Palpable tender areas of dysfunction, which often display measurable changes of cutaneous electrical potential, may be regarded as common to all these systems.

Neuro-muscular Technique (NMT) is a method of diagnostic and therapeutic value, which is simple in its application yet has enormous potential. The developer of this technique was Stanley Lief who was born in Lutzen in the Baltic state of Latvia in the early 1890s. He was one of the five children of Isaac and Riva Lief (Riva was the author's grandfather's eldest sister). The family emigrated to South Africa in the early 1900s where Stanley was given a basic primary school education before starting work in his father's trading store in Roodeport, Transvaal.

His health was poor and this led to an interest in physical culture, one source of inspiration for which was in the form of magazines from America. Eventually he worked his passage to

Stanley Lief

the U.S.A. in order to train under the legendary Bernarr Macfadden. He qualified in chiropractic and naturopathy before the First World War, and was in Britain at the outbreak of war. After serving in the army during the war he returned to England and worked in institutional Nature Cure resorts until 1925 when he established his own Hydro, Champneys, at Tring in Hertfordshire.

At this world-famous healing resort he established his reputation as a daring and pioneering healer. By using the dietetic, fasting, hydrotherapeutic and physical methods, by which means naturopathy aims to restore normality to the sick body, he developed a huge following. During his most successful years before the Second World War he evolved the technique which this book attempts to describe.

Boris Chaitow

Stanley Lief and his cousin Boris Chaitow, who worked as his assistant at Champneys before and during the Second World War, developed and refined the uses of NMT. Boris Chaitow was also born in Latvia and as a child went to live in South Africa. He was qualified as a lawyer and was in practice with my father when he became inspired by Stanley Lief's example and, with Lief's help, trained in America before joining him at Champneys in 1937. Boris Chaitow is still in practice at his superb health resort in the Cape, South Africa.

In this book the basic application, together with some specialized soft tissue manipulation techniques, will be presented, as will various reflex systems which fall within the scope of soft tissue treatment in general and NMT in particular. Detailed reference to and illustrations of the neurolymphatic reflexes of Chapman, together with illustrations of other reflex patterns such as myofascial trigger points, have therefore been included.

NMT, as a modality, may be incorporated into any system of physical medicine. It may (and indeed often should) be used as a treatment on its own, or it may accompany (preceding for preference) manipulative and other physical modalities. Its main use up to the present has been in the hands (literally) of the osteopathic profession. However, those physiotherapists, chiropractors and doctors of physical medicine who have studied and used NMT have found it complementary to their own methods of practice.

I firmly believe that this method, if comprehended and used as Stanley Lief and Boris Chaitow intended, can substantially aid practitioners in resolving the problems of many of their patients. Since it offers a simultaneous diagnostic and therapeutic capability NMT is time saving, energy saving and, above all, efficient.

The specialized soft tissue manipulative methods described may be used independently or as part of NMT treatment. Practice is required in all these methods, and the key to the successful use of NMT is the ability to sense accurately what it is that the hands are feeling, together with having a clear picture of what the particular movement or technique being employed is aimed at achieving. If the practitioner can learn to 'see' with his hands, and by using them let the patient's body 'tell its own tale', then the intelligent application of the methods described here will provide a major step towards the recovery of health.

Holistic methods of healing demand that in order to create the situation for the maintenance or the restoration of health the individual must be seen as a totality. It is necessary, therefore, to recognize all the various factors affecting both the internal and external environment of the individual as being part of the complex interacting totality which can influence the individual for good or ill. In the end the body is self-healing, self-repairing and self-maintaining, if the pre-requisites for health are present. Emotional stability, nutritional balance, hygienic considerations all play their parts, as does the structural and mechanical integrity of the body.

No method that is worthy of consideration as part of the therapeutic resources of practitioners conscious of the holistic approach should have undesirable side-effects. Nothing that is done to the body in the name of therapeutic endeavour should detract from the body's ability to function normally and efficiently. NMT, which aims at restoring structural and functional integrity to the musculoskeletal component of the body is safe and efficient and produces no adverse reactions or effects if used correctly.

NMT takes its place as part of the armamentary of all those who seek to aid the healing capacity of the body. In setting down the methods employed in NMT the author is acutely aware of the limitations of the written word in conveying the essence of such techniques. The illustrations provide a further aid, but nothing can take the place of individual instruction. It is to be hoped that courses and seminars will continue to provide the opportunity for practitioners to learn, at first hand, the scope of these methods. This book should aid such study as it provides the practitioners or student with the raw material with which to begin the study of an invaluable technique.

Chapter 1

Somatic Dysfunction—
the Soft Tissue Component

The soft tissues of the body are the source of a great deal of pain and dysfunction. This pain can be localized or general and it can also be referred or reflex in nature. Terminology applied to soft tissue lesions and problems is not always accurate. Such terms as 'fibrositis' and 'muscular rheumatism' do not necessarily indicate anything at all in a clinical sense. Such expressions as 'stringy', 'nodular', 'indurated' etc. are also inexact.

They do, however, describe what the practitioner's hands feel and, as such, have a subjective value. But, for the purpose of accuracy, a comprehensive term can be applied to all lesions of the musculo-skeletal system. This term is 'somatic dysfunction' and it can be defined as impaired or altered function of related components of the somatic (body framework) system, i.e. skeletal, arthrodial, and myofascial structures and related vascular, lymphatic, and neural elements.

This general expression (somatic dysfunction) obviously requires specific definition in any given case and this should include identification of the particular structure, tissue or area involved. The soft tissues of the body have specific interrelated functions to perform. A variety of factors can contribute to local or general dysfunction of traumatic, postural, pathological or psychological origin. Such dysfunction might itself become the source of referred pain and other symptoms.

Some of the various components which might contribute towards somatic dysfunction and the ramifications thereof will be considered, as will several therapeutic techniques which aim at normalizing the soft tissues and the reflex end-products of somatic dysfunction. A number of researchers in this field have examined different aspects of the causes of soft tissue dysfunction and it will be advantageous to examine some of the findings and theories which have resulted, as well as their solutions.

Sixty per cent of the mass of the body comprises the musculo-skeletal system. There is structural and functional continuity between all the hard and soft tissues which make up this mechanical component of the human machine. The tendency to think of a local lesion as existing in isolation should be discouraged and an awareness should be cultivated of the interrelated nature of this assortment of tissues. The musculo-skeletal system consists of muscles, ligaments, tendons, bones and fascia (connective tissue) and is the main consumer of body energy. Apart from its obvious role in the support and motion of the body it is involved in biochemical and biomechanical activities.

The Fascia The fascia is of great significance in its role of supporting and providing cohesion to the body structures. Its functions are varied and complex and include the following:

1. Connective tissue provides a supporting matrix for more highly organized structures.

2. Because it contains mesenchymal cells of an embryonic type, connective tissue provides a generalized tissue capable of giving rise, under certain circumstances, to more specialized elements.

3. It provides, by its fascial planes, pathways for nerves, and lymphatic vessels.

4. It supplies restraining mechanisms by the differentiation of retention bands, fibrous pulleys, check ligaments, etc.

5. Where connective tissue is loose in texture it allows movement between adjacent structures and, by the formation of bursal sacs, it reduces the effects of pressure and friction.

6. Deep fascia ensheaths and preserves the characteristic contour of the limbs, and promotes the circulation in the veins and lymphatic vessels.

7. The superficial fascia, which forms the panniculus adiposus, allows for the storage of fat and also provides a surface covering which aids in the conservation of body heat.

8. By virtue of its fibroplastic activity, connective tissue aids in the repair of injuries by the deposition of collagenous fibres (scar tissue).

9. The ensheathing layer of deep fascia, as well as intermuscular septa and interosseous membranes, provides additional surface areas for muscular attachment.

10. The meshes of loose connective tissue contain the 'tissue fluid'; they provide an essential medium through which the cellular elements of other tissues are brought into functional relation with blood and lymph. Connective tissue has a nutritive function.

11. The histiocytes of connective tissue comprise part of an important defence mechanism against bacterial invasion by their phagocytic activity. They also play a part as scavengers in removing cell debris and foreign material.

12. Connective tissue represents an important 'neutralizer' or detoxicator to both endogenous toxins (those produced under physiological conditions), and exogenous toxins (those which are introduced from outside the organism). Much of this neutralizing or detoxicating function appears to be associated with reactions at the surface of the numerous fibres.

These, then, represent the major functions of this ubiquitous, tenacious connective tissue which is a living tissue deeply involved in the fundamental processes of the body's metabolism.

Modern techniques of electron and phase microscopy have been used to study myofascial biochemistry activity. Much of the fascia and connective tissue is made of tubular structures. Erlinghauser[1] has shown that lymph and cerebro-spinal fluid spreads throughout the body via these channels. The implications of this knowledge have not yet been fully realized or investigated by physiologists.

Selye[2] called stress the non-specific element in disease production. In describing the relationship between the General Adaptation Syndrome (GAS)—i.e. alarm reaction, resistance phase, exhaustion—and the Local Adaptation Syndrome (LAS), Selye emphasized the importance of connective tissue. He indicated that stress results in a pattern of adaptation, individual to each organism.   **GAS and LAS**

In assessing the patient the neuro-muscular-skeletal changes represent a record of the attempts on the part of the body to adapt and adjust to the stresses imposed upon it. The repeated postural and traumatic insults of a lifetime, combined with the tensions of emotional and psychological origin, will often present a confusing pattern of tense, contracted, bunched, fatigued fibrous tissue.

The minutiae of the process are not for the moment at issue. What is important is the realization that, due to prolonged stress of a postural, psychic or mechanical type, a discrete area of the body will become so altered by its efforts to compensate and adapt to this stress, that structural and, eventually, pathological changes will become apparent. Other researchers have shown that the type of stress involved can be entirely physical in nature (e.g. repetitive postural strain such as that adopted by a dentist or hairdresser), or purely psychic in nature (e.g. chronic repressed anger).

More often than not a combination of mental and physical stresses will so alter neuro-muscular-skeletal structures as to create an identifiable physical change, which will itself be a generator of further stress, such as pain, joint restriction, general discomfort and fatigue. Such changes can also be the result of traumatic episodes and one could have either chronic or acute lesions which in all respects duplicate each other, apart from the long-term tissue changes which would be manifest in the chronic lesion.

When an individual is conscious of being in danger, real or imagined, the total organism is involved and the homeostatic mechanism is activated to protect itself from danger. The chronic stress pattern that can result in the total organism will produce long-term muscular contraction. This in turn, if prolonged, will have profound effects on, for example, the cardio-vascular system. Even simple muscular contraction of the arm, if sustained, will elevate blood pressure by 10mm to 20mm Hg.[3] Jacobson[4] stated:

> Physiological studies indicate beyond reasonable doubt that, with or without attendant emotion, neuro-muscular hyperkinesis is characteristic of over-energetic living and, in consequence, the heart overworks protractedly with resultant wear and tear, manifested in diversified cardiac pathology.

The ramifications of neuro-muscular stress are therefore more widespread than the simple pain and discomfort level. Energy loss, mechanical inefficiency, pain, cardio-vascular pathology, hypertension etc., all are a possible result of neuro-muscular dysfunction and are therefore amenable to correction by whatever means will normalize this dysfunction.

The tissues which we are concerned with and some of the changes that occur in them will be considered later in the book. At this stage, however, it is necessary to establish beyond reasonable doubt that soft tissues of the musculoskeletal system, when subjected to acute or chronic embarrassment, will change and adapt themselves in a predictable manner. This adaptation will be seen almost always to be at the expense of optimum functional ability. Such changes will also be seen to be the on-going source of further physiological embarrassment. Finally it will be seen that removal of such changes or lesions or dysfunctions is frequently possible.

Our concern in this work is with the soft tissue component of such processes. As such there is a large degree of overlapping of interest with the practitioner whose prime interest in restoring structural integrity focuses more on the bony structures of the body. Manipulative therapists, physiotherapists, chiropractors and osteopaths all use techniques to attempt to normalize positional and motional disturbances within the body framework. To some extent all take into account the soft tissues when assessing and correcting such problems. The aim of this book is to emphasize the importance of the soft tissue component. From the therapeutic viewpoint a specific technique for the alleviation of the soft tissue aspect of such problems will be seen at times to obviate the necessity for joint manipulation.

Stress Responses

Stress responses[5] on the part of the body have been divided into four general areas of consideration. All or some of these factors can be present in any given case.

Physiological. This might involve general overall muscle tension of a postural nature or specific localized tension resulting from particular over-use of a part (typists, dentists, tailors, etc.).

Emotional. All emotional changes are mirrored in muscular changes. Emotional attitudes, such as anger or fear, as well as moods such as excitement or depression, all produce muscular postures and patterns. There is a close relationship between habitual tension patterns and postures, and psychological attitudes and conflicts.

Behavioural. All movement requires muscular activity. Certain patterns of use establish themselves. Often individual awareness of the pattern of use is diminished and habitually repetitive actions take place with resultant muscular hypertension. .

Structural. Muscle tissue will change in texture, chemistry, tone etc. and will also modify and alter the framework of the body, warping and cramping its potential for normal use. The body will be bent and distorted to meet the stresses imposed from without and within.

Barlow, whose work follows that of Alexander,[6] suggests that there exists a self-regulating tendency in muscular behaviour. The term 'postural homeo-stasis' implies a return to a balanced resting state after activity. Such regulation is usually at an unconscious level. He gives the example of a patient with persistent low back pain who, in the resting position, demonstrates a particular set of muscular distortions such as tense erector spina on the left and a tense trapezius on the right, together with a pelvic twist to the right. On activity all these spasms become accentuated.

This demonstrates a residual tension pattern which has never been resolved. This, Barlow suggests, can be normalized by restoring a 'balanced resting state'. It might be, however, only partially released through treatment which only deals with part of the causative components. In such a case activity or stress would reactivate the whole pattern of imbalance. In this suggested restoration of homoeostatic equilibrium Barlow would, of course, employ postural re-education of the individual. I would contend that greater success would be achieved by the use of soft tissue normalization, through neuro-muscular treatment and possibly manipulation, combined with such re-education.

Where pain exists in tense musculature, Barlow suggests that in the absence of other pathology such pain results from: **Source of Pain**

1. The muscle itself through some noxious metabolic product (this has been called 'Factor P'[7]) or an interference in blood circulation due to spasm, resulting in relative ischaemia.

2. The muscular insertion into the periosteum, such as that caused by an actual lifting of the periosteal tissue by marked, or repetitive, muscular tension (e.g. 'tennis elbow').

3. The joint involved, which can become restricted and over-approximated. In advanced cases osteo-arthritic changes can result from the repeated microtrauma of repeated muscular misuse. Many chronic joint conditions are preventable if early muscular stress patterns are spotted and normalized prior to such damage taking place.

4. Nerve irritation, which can be produced spinally or along the course of the nerve as a result of chronic muscular contractions. These can produce disc and general spinal mechanical faults, with all that that can lead to.

5. Variations in pain threshold will make all these factors more or less significant and obvious.

Where pain has been produced by repetitive habits, postural and otherwise, with emotional and psychological overtones, the task of the therapist is complex indeed. It is certainly true that tension can be partially released or relaxed without resolving the underlying pattern. This must be avoided if repeated recurrence of painful episodes is to be minimized. What must be aimed at is a state of relative equilibrium of body structure and function.

Reich[8] outlined an understanding of the postures and defensive tensions produced by neurotic patients. He showed that such individuals often behaved as though they were 'half-dead'. Their normal functioning, on all levels, was diminished and restricted. 'They were disturbed sexually, they were disturbed in their work function, their bodily processes lacked rhythm, their breathing was uncoordinated'[9].

Reich and his followers have demonstrated the capability of emotions to mobilize or paralyse the body. Continued and repeated stress is shown to produce 'blockages' and restrictions in the musculoskeletal system which, if unreleased, become self-perpetuating and are themselves the source of pain and further stress. The ability to relax is lost and the drain on nervous energy is profound.

Neurosis would seem to be the disease of modern times. The bioenergetic answer to this problem is to aid in the release of these tensions by a complex set of exercises, including facial expressions and body positions, accompanied by breathing techniques. These methods are doubtless successful in many cases, but do not concern our present study. What is important is the realization that neuro-muscular restriction, as evidenced by stiff body use, may often be a manifestation of deep psychological and emotional stress. Its release, by whatever means, can be seen to be a desirable step in the restoration of normality.

Tissue Changes   Taylor[10] has postulated that the tissue changes, apparent to the trained palpating hand, often result from changes in the thermo-dynamic equilibrium. He states that the body is a thermo-dynamic system and, as such, the alterations in the extracellular fluids, viscosity, pH, electrophoretic changes, colloidal osmotic pressure, etc. are subject to thermo-dynamic laws. One of these states that the total energy of such a system and its surroundings must remain constant, though the energy may be changed from one to another due to alterations of the stresses imposed. Through postural misuse and gravitational effects, particular changes would result in energy loss and therefore stasis and stagnation in the fascia involved. One of the phenomena of thermo-dynamics is that of thixotropy in which gels become more solid with energy loss and more fluid with energy input. Such changes are certainly palpable in soft tissues before and after neuro-muscular treatment.

Taylor has stated that manipulative pressure and stretching are the most effective ways of modifying energy potentials of abnormal soft tissues. Little[11] believes that an additional beneficial effect results from the interaction of the bio-energy mechanism of the practitioner and the bio-energy field of the patient.

Eeman[12] has shown that after each simple movement that we perform we retain a degree of unconscious contractive muscular activity. This unconscious continuation of objective contraction is not only wasteful of energy but productive of long-term changes within the tissues involved.

He has further shown that unless, and until, neuro-muscular relaxation is achieved there cannot be a total resting state of the mind. Over and above the important factors of posture, functional ability and pain the musculoskeletal element is seen to play a vital role in the conservation, or otherwise, of energy and in the attainment, or otherwise, of a truly relaxed mind. Whilst the origins of musculo-skeletal tensions can be either psychic or physical their continuity ensures a constant degree of psychic stress as a feedback from this tension.

Rolfing   Rolf[13] suggests that the human organism as an energy mass is subject to gravitational law. As a plastic medium, capable of change, Rolfing attempts to reorganize and balance the body in relation to gravitational forces. This is done by using pressure and stretch techniques on the fascial tissues in a precise sequence of body areas. The beneficial effects are claimed to be physical, emotional, postural and behavioural.

Rolf states:

Our ignorance of the role and significance of fascia is profound. Therefore even in theory it is easy to overlook the possibility that far-reaching changes may be made not only in structural contour, but also in functional manifestation, through better organization of the layer of superficial fascia which enwraps the body. Experiment demonstrates that drastic changes may be made in the body, solely by stretching, separating and relaxing superficial fascia in an appropriate manner.

Osteopathic manipulators have observed and recorded the extent to which all degenerative change in the body, be it muscular, nervous, circulatory or organic, reflects in superficial fascia. Any degree of degeneration, however minor, changes the bulk of the fascia, modifies its thickness and draws it into ridges in areas overlying deeper tensions and rigidities. Conversely, as this elastic envelope is stretched, manipulative mechanical energy is added to it, and the fascial colloid becomes more 'sol' and less 'gel'. The biophysics of this process has been discussed in a classical paper by R. B. Taylor.[14] As a result of the added energy, as well as of a directional contribution in applying it, the underlying structures, including the muscles which determine the placement of the body parts in space, and also their relations to each other, have come a little closer to the normal. ('Normal' as used here must be differentiated from 'average'.) The patient feels 'so much better'.

Gutstein[15] seeks to denote localized functional sensory and/or motor abnormalities of musculoskeletal tissue (comprising muscle, fascia, tendon, bone and joint) as myodysneuria. He sees the causes of such changes as multiple and among these are:

(a) Acute and chronic infections which it is postulated stimulate sympathetic nerve activity via their toxins.

(b) Excessive heat or cold, changes in atmospheric pressure and draughts.

(c) Mechanical injuries, both major and repeated minor micro-traumas. Postural strain, unaccustomed exercises etc., which may predispose towards future changes by lowering the threshold for future stimuli.

(d) Allergic and endocrine factors which can cause imbalance in the autonomic nervous system.

(e) Inherited factors making adjustment to environmental factors difficult.

(f) Arthritic changes: since muscles are the active components of the musculoskeletal system it is logical to assume that their circulatory state has influence over bones and joints. Spasm in muscle may contribute towards osteoarthritic changes and such changes may produce further neuro-muscular changes which themselves produce symptoms.

(g) Visceral diseases may intensify and precipitate somatic symptoms in the distribution of their spinal and adjacent segments.

Diagnosis of myodysneuria is made according to some of the following criteria:

(a) A varying degree of muscular tension and contraction is usually present although sometimes adjacent, non-indurated tissue is more painful.

(b) Sensitivity to pressure or palpation of affected muscles and their adjuncts.

Marked contraction may require the application of deep pressure to demonstrate tenderness.

Pathophysiology The changes which occur in tissue involved in the onset of myodysneuria, according to Gutstein, are thought to be initiated by localized sympathetic predominance, associated with changes in the hydrogen ion concentration and calcium and sodium balance in the tissue fluids.[16] This is associated with vaso-constriction and hypoxia. Pain results, it is thought, by these alterations affecting the pain sensors and proprioceptors. Muscle spasm and hard nodular localized tetanic contractions of muscle bundles[17] together with vasomotor and musculomotor stimulation intensify each other, creating a vicious cycle of self-perpetuating impulses. There are varied and complex patterns of referred symptoms which may result from such 'trigger' areas as well as local pain and minor disturbances.

Such sensations as aching, soreness, tenderness, heaviness and tiredness may all be manifest as may modification of muscular activity due to contraction resulting in tightness, stiffness, swelling etc.

Cathie[18] maintains that the contractive phase of fascial activity supercedes all other qualities of fascia. The attachments of fascia he states have a tendency to shorten after periods of marked activity which are followed by periods of inactivity and the ligaments become tighter and thicker with advancing age. The properties of fascia (connective tissue) that he regards as being important to therapeutic consideration are listed as being that:

1. It is richly endowed with nerve endings.
2. It has the ability to contract and to stretch elastically.
3. It gives extensive muscular attachment.
4. It supports and stabilizes, thus enhancing the postural balance of the body.
5. It is vitally involved in all aspects of motion.
6. It aids in circulatory economy, especially of venous and lymphatic fluids.
7. Fascial change will precede many of the chronic degenerative diseases.
8. Fascial changes predispose towards chronic tissue congestion.
9. Such chronic passive congestion precedes the formation of fibrous tissue which then proceeds to an increase in hydrogen ion concentration of articular and periarticular structures.
10. Fascial specializations produce definite stress bands.
11. Sudden stress (trauma) on fascial tissue will often result in a burning type of pain.
12. Fascia is a major arena of inflammatory processes.
13. Fluids and infectious processes often travel along fascial planes.
14. The CNS is surrounded by fascial tissue (dura mater) which in the skull attaches to bone. Dysfunction in these tissues can have profound and widespread effects.

Changes which occur in connective tissue, and which result in such alterations as thickening, shortening, calcification and erosion, may be a result of sudden or sustained tension or traction. Cathie points out that many 'trigger spots' correspond to points where nerves pierce fascial investments. The causes of derangement may therefore be seen to result from faulty muscular activity, alteration in bony relationships, visceral positional change (e.g. visceroptosis) and the use of unnatural positions. All these can be sustained, repetitive causes or single, violently induced changes. Chemical (nutritional) factors must also be considered.

As Pauling[19] points out:

> Many of the results of deprivation of ascorbic acid involve a deficiency in connective tissue. Connective tissue is largely responsible for the strength of bones, teeth, skin, of the body. It consists of the fibrous protein collagen.

He goes on to point out that in deficiency of Vitamin C this binding material becomes less efficient and more fluid. Pauling concludes that the effectiveness of Vitamin C in helping the body contain virus particles may to some extent be a result of its strengthening action on connective tissue, which would impede the motion of virus particles through tissue. This illustrates again the ubiquitous nature of the musculoskeletal tissues in general and fascia in particular and the profound effect on the body economy of dysfunction in any of its myriad components.

Cyriax[20] believes that all primary 'fibrositic' conditions are a result of articular **Fibrositis** lesions (dysfunctions). A secondary fibrositic change may result, he states, from traumatic injury to soft tissues (e.g. capsular adhesion at the shoulder after injury) which should be called fibrosis, not fibrositis. This he sees as scar tissue formation. Other secondary fibrositic conditions can result from rheumatoid disease, infection (such as epidemic myalgia) and parasitic infection (*triclina spiralis*). All other muscular and soft tissue dysfunctions Cyriax regards as a result of joint dysfunction which can then produce muscular protective spasm, muscular wasting, pain etc., and which can only be normalized, he maintains, by correction of the joint lesion. Neuro-muscular theory and practice show that appropriate normalization of the soft tissues can often achieve joint normalization without active manipulative treatment of such a joint.

Cyriax does point out that fibrous tissue is capable of maintaining inflammation, originally traumatic, almost as a matter of habit. In such cases he opts for hydrocortisone injections as the appropriate measure to 'break' this habit. Such treatment can work, but all too often fails as underlying mechanical dysfunction has not been normalized.

Stoddard[21] in discussing contracted musculature, describes its 'stringy' feel resulting from the continuous contraction of some muscle fibres and, like Cyriax ascribes the cause to the underlying joint dysfunctions. The resulting ache and pain is usually a result of circulatory embarrassment as metabolic wastes build-up due to sustained muscular contraction. Muscular guarding is always seen to indicate deeper pathological changes (e.g. T.B. spine, osteomyelitis, disc herniation etc.).

Stoddard sees the metabolic wastes, which may result from a degree of stasis, as causing a vicious cycle in perpetuating muscular contraction, leading eventually to fibrous changes occuring. There is no indication that Stoddard considers such changes to be of primary importance in his treatment programme. He does stress the importance of exercises to strengthen muscle groups and of correct posture, but does not indicate any great interest in treatment of the soft tissue themselves.

Connective Tissue Massage

A system which does concentrate on the soft tissues is Connective Tissue Massage. This is a soft tissue system of German origin which has marked similarities to Neuro-muscular Technique. Maria Ebner[22] describes its principles as follows:

Principles of application. The autonomic nervous system serves to co-ordinate the various structures of the human body. The structures under autonomic control continue to function as long as the body is alive, and are independent of voluntary control. The severance of a somatic spinal nerve will absolish the function of the organ which it supplies. The severance of an autonomic nerve will not interfere with the function of the supplied organ during the resting state. The heart with all autonomic connections severed will continue to beat, provided its nourishment is maintained. The impulse for its basic function arises in the organ itself. The function of the autonomic nervous system is to co-ordinate the various structures and make them adaptable to varying and changing stimuli arising from changes in the environment. The autonomic centres serve to modify the reaction to peripheral stimuli of somatic and autonomic origin, and establish harmonious interaction of structures under somatic and autonomic control, e.g., thermal stimuli registered by the terminal somatic nerves will cause adaptive constriction or dilatation of peripheral blood vessels. The close interrelation between the somatic, autonomic and endocrine systems makes it impossible for pathological changes to take place in any one structure without causing adaptive changes in other structures. Surface changes relating to sensibility and contour in organic pathological disturbances have already been reported by Head in 1898.

Capillary changes in skin segments within the dermatome supply of a pathologically affected organ have been investigated microscopically by Dittmar (1943) and by Rouanet (1946).

Changes in muscular tension and pain sensibility have been discussed by Mackenzie (1917) and others. The most universally known example is the circumscribed abdominal tension in appendicitis.

The pathway responsible for peripheral changes in pathological organic disturbances may also be responsible for changes in the opposite direction. Hartman (1928) describes changes in connective tissue within the dermatomes of the heart, causing heart symptoms and clearing up after treatment of the peripheral connective tissue.

Nonnenbruch and Gross (1952) describe similar phenomena which they investigated. These observations should prove that body surface, organs and connective tissue within the segmental nerve supply are connected by reflex pathways. Changes in one part of the segment may be responsible for alteration in other parts of the segmental supply. The previously described distribution of autonomic cell stations and fibres will have made it clear that tissue changes due to alteration in blood supply will not remain confined to one particular segment. Treatment of peripheral changes should therefore be continued until the circulation over the whole body surface is normalized to the greatest possible extent. Hypersensitive zones must disappear before terminating the treatment.

Pathways concerned may be as follows, choosing stomach pathology as an example. The stomach is supplied by the great splanchnic nerve which derives its fibres from the segments T.5 to 9. Ascending sympathetic branches pass to cervical ganglia from the same segments. Maximal points for stomach pathology lie in the dermatomes of C.3 to T.5 to 9.

Viscero-cutaneous. Afferent from stomach—Posterior Root Ganglion (PRG)—lateral horn cell white ramus—sympathetic ganglion—grey ramus—somatic nerve carrying fibres to blood vessels.

Result. Vasoconstriction in the periphery and hyperaesthesia. Changes in subcutaneous tissue.

Cutaneo-visceral. Altered tension in the periphery registered by posterior afferent—PRG—lateral horn—sympathetic ganglion—postganglionic fibre to stomach.

Result. Interference with stomach blood supply and new flare-up. The peripheral changes are invariably present but usually clear up within two to three weeks. For unknown reasons they sometimes do not clear up and cause new flare-up.

Viscero-motor. This is a variation of the viscero-cutaneous effect, except that the connector fibre establishes a relay into the anterior horn. The new fibre carries excitatory impulses to muscles within the segmental supply.

Result. Alteration in muscle tension.

The treatment itself employs pulling and stretching of the various soft tissues of the body in a precise manner. Such 'strokes' are both diagnostic and therapeutic, having both local and distal reflex effects. This is in common with Neuro-muscular Technique.

R. L. Nimmo[23] described his system for normalizing body structures as one which detected and eliminated noxious 'points' which generate reflex effects; eliminated hypertonia and hypotonia in muscles to enable restoration of bony normality; and corrected abnormalities in ligaments and tendons. The sensitive points generating noxious stimuli result, according to Nimmo, from repetitive irritation resulting from facilitation. Travell, Mennell and others have worked in this field and some of their therapeutic ideas will be discussed later. At this point it would be advantageous to examine that aspect of body function which has been so closely investigated by Korr, the great osteopathic researcher and theoretician.

Korr[24] states:

> The spinal cord is the keyboard on which the brain plays when it calls for activity or for change in activity. But each 'key' in the console sounds, not an individual 'tone', such as the contraction of a particular group of muscle fibres, but a whole 'melody' of activity, even a 'symphony' of motion. In other words, built into the cord is a large repertoire of patterns of activity, each involving the complex, harmonious, delicately balanced orchestration of the contractions and relaxations of many muscles. The brain 'thinks' in terms of whole motions, not individual muscles. It calls selectively, for the preprogrammed patterns in the cord and brain stem, modifying them in countless ways and combining them in an infinite variety of still more complex patterns. Each activity is also subject to further modulation, refinement, and adjustment by the afferent feedback continually streaming in from the participating muscles, tendons, and joints.

Professor Michael Patterson[25] explains the theory of facilitation as follows:

Theory of Facilitation

> The concept of the facilitated segment states that because of abnormal afferent or sensory inputs to a particular area of the spinal cord, that area is kept in a state of constant increased excitation. This facilitation allows normally ineffectual or subliminal stimuli to become effective in producing efferent output from the facilitated segment, causing both skeletal and visceral organs innervated by the affected segment to be maintained in a state of overactivity. It is probable that the 'osteopathic lesion', or somatic dysfunction with which a facilitated segment is

associated, is the direct result of the abnormal segmental activity as well as being partially responsible for the facilitation.

Although the effects of the facilitated segment on various skeletal and visceral functions are well documentated, little is understood about the genesis and maintenance of spinal facilitation. Even the question of why some traumas cause facilitation and others do not remain unanswered.

The concept of the facilitated segment is essentially that abnormal or altered inputs from a source of irritation impinging on the spinal cord will keep the interneurons or motoneurons of that spinal segment in a constant state of excitement, thus allowing normally ineffectual inputs to produce outputs to all organs receiving innervation from the excited area. This concept implies that the spinal cord is a relatively passive mediator of the influences imposed on it and that the neural paths act as communicators of that activity.

The recent research on spinal functions seems to indicate, however, that the spinal cord, besides being the determiner of where abnormal activity is sent by virtue of predetermined pathways, may participate actively in either controlling abnormal or unusually intense inputs or amplifying and retaining such inputs in certain circumstances.

Initially, only intensities of afferent input above a certain level would result in increased sensitivity of the spinal pathway. Inputs of lower intensity either would cause no alterations or would cause an actual decrease in sensitivity as a protective mechanism against undue changes in homeostatic mechanisms. It is apparent that the potential for sensitization by different types of afferent inputs may differ widely. Thus, inputs from pain receptors may sensitize the pathway at low levels because of the properties of the initial synapses between pain afferent fibres and interneurons. In this event an initially protective increase in response might occur, but a detrimental facilitation of a segment would follow. On the other hand, inputs from joint receptors have a less dramatic effect at similar input levels.

The model also permits the prediction that emotional arousal would affect the susceptibility of the pathways to sensitization. The increase in descending influences from the emotionally aroused subject would result in an increase in toxic excitement in the pathways and allow all additional inputs to produce sensitization at low intensities. Thus, highly emotional persons or those in a highly emotional situation would be expected to show a higher incidence of facilitation of spinal pathways. Since the higher brain centres do influence the tonic levels of the spinal paths, it might be expected also that physical training and mental attitudes would tend to alter the tonic excitability as well, reducing the person's susceptibility to sensitization from everyday stress. Thus the athlete would be expected to withstand a comparatively high level of afferent input prior to experiencing the self-perpetuating results of sensitization.

A further corollary of the hypothesis is that slowly developing conditions or slowly increasing inputs would result in less sensitization at high levels than sudden inputs. The slowly developing of chronic source of increased sensory input initially would cause habituation, resulting in resistance to sensitization until the input level was abnormally high. On the other hand, sudden increases in input, such as a sudden postural stress, would be expected to produce sensitization of the neural pathways most rapidly.

The hypothesis presented here explains a phenomenon observed in clinical practice and described by Jones in 1964. He termed it 'spontaneous release by positioning'. Jones outlined a procedure developed to reduce somatic dysfunction in several apparently severe cases. He noted that a patient with a severe lesion which was interfering with normal movement and function gained considerable relief from the lesion if he was positioned in such a way that the discomfort was stopped. Although placing the patient in such a position of comfort apparently required heroic positioning at times, holding the patient in the exaggerated position for at least 90 seconds often allowed a return to normal posture and activity with no recurrence of the symptoms. It would be assumed from the model that the sensitization caused by the constant pain inputs from the affected area would drop below a critical level during the period of pain cessation. A corollary to the decrease in sensitization over time would be that for a time following the aforementioned treatment, the patient would be highly liable to recurrence of the problems as a result of residual sensitization and the long-lasting effects of conditioning of the abnormal activity. This liability would be gradually reversed by normal inputs and responses. It would also be expected that highly nervous persons might require a longer period in a position of comfort to achieve relief and that such persons would remain vulnerable for longer periods to reacquisition of sensitization or facilitation than would less emotional patients. A closely allied aspect of the sensitization concept is that a relatively minor increase in sensitization which might be caused during daily activity could be corrected during sleep as a result of the decrease in descending activity and the accompanying muscular relaxation. Thus, besides the damping effects of habituation, normal relaxation should tend to relieve minor segmental problems which otherwise might become increasingly acute. However, it will also be expected that drugs often used to relieve somatic dysfunction, such as muscle relaxants or central nervous system depressants would be successful only if a sufficient degree of relaxation or decrease in the overactive sensory input could be achieved. It is possible that often such drugs do not work because of increased inputs from visceral and non-muscular tissues which remain a source of high afferent bombardment.

The application of high-velocity and muscle energy manipulative techniques to the somatic dysfunction remains the most effective means of treating these disorders. In a brilliant recent article, Korr proposed a mechanism involving the gamma motor system and muscle proprioceptors as one of the common causes of sustained muscle contraction associated with the somatic dysfunction. He proposed that manipulative procedures involving high-velocity, short-amplitude forces as well as muscle energy techniques would act to force the central nervous system to correct abnormally high excitation of the muscle spindles and allow the muscle to return to its normal length and the joint to its normal motion. Similar reasoning with regard to decreasing the spindle activity would apply to functional techniques, which, instead of forcing a contracted muscle against its contraction, would allow it to continue to shorten until relaxed normally. In any of these procedures afferent input to the cord would be reduced for a sufficient time to allow the sensitization to decrease below the critical level. That is, afferent input would be reduced either directly or via central brain influences, to a level below that required to sustain sensitization.

In 1948 Korr stated that:

1. The body is a unit; all parts function in the context of the entire organism.
2. Disease is a reaction of the organism as a whole. Abnormal structure or function in one part exerts abnormal influence on other parts and, therefore, on the total body economy.
3. The organism has the inherent capacity to defend itself, to repair itself, and to resist serious upsets in equilibria.
4. The nervous system plays a dominant organizing role in the disease processes.
5. There is a somatic component to every disease which is not only a manifestation of the disease, *but an important contributing factor.*
6. Appropriate treatment of the somatic component has important therapeutic value in that it leads to improvement in the other components.

The consensus of opinion would seem to indicate that the neuro-muscular component of joint dysfunction is of importance in both the production and maintenance of the problems. Its normalization can remove a major contributory factor to the affected joint and can further be of value by removing the site of trigger points whose ramifications can affect the body adversely in numerous ways. Postural integrity and a reasonable level of relaxation are also dependent upon neuro-muscular tonus being normal. The correction of joint dysfunction by manipulation or exercise may be speeded up by soft-tissue correction as can maintenance of the affected area in an improved state of functional integrity.

Stanley Lief Neuro-muscular Technique (NMT) is a system that has evolved over the past forty years from the original work of the late Stanley Lief. Lief was a pioneering and gifted practitioner of manipulative therapy. As a trained chiropractor and osteopath he was aware of the need for a means by which soft-tissue structures could be prepared for subsequent manipulation. In the 1930s he studied the work of Rabagliatti whose work *Initis* influenced his work towards dealing with connective tissue problems. He also studied the work of a practitioner of Hindu manipulation Dewanchand Varma who was practising in Paris. Varma used a system called 'Pranotherapy' and in his book *The Human Machine and Its Forces* (London, 1938) he states:

> We have discovered that the circulation of the nervous currents, slows down occasionally because of the obstruction caused by adhesions; the muscular fibres harden and the nervous currents can no longer pass through them. We have demonstrated effective and positive methods designed to restore nervous equilibrium which promotes the healthy circulation of blood, so that new tissues begin to be built up, again. Our method of treatment, by the removal of all obstacles to the flow of nervous current, allows energy to proceed unimpeded.

Lief found various techniques of Varma useful and out of these ideas and methods developed his own soft tissue method—NMT. His cousin Boris Chaitow D.C., who worked with Lief during this period, describes the early development of NMT as follows:[26]

> In the middle of the 1930s Stanley Lief realized that the integrity of a joint was to a great extent related to the character of the tissues surrounding the joint, related to muscle, tendons, ligaments, blood and nerve supply etc. He felt that in order the better to achieve effective mobility and integrity of function of joints—particularly in the spine but also in *all* bony articular relationships—it was advisable to normalize, as best one could, the adjacent soft tissues by removing any function-interfering factors, such as tensions, contractions, adhesions, spasms, fibrositic contractures etc., with appropriate use of fingers and hands to those tissues. To this end the neuro-muscular technique was evolved to cover *every* possible type of lesion in *whatever* part of the body (articular, soft tissue, abdominal, glandular, nervous, vascular etc.).
>
> It so happened that at that particular time Stanley Lief had heard of a well-known Indian practitioner named Varma operating in Paris, who was applying an unusual but very effective soft-tissue technique on patients with remarkable benefits. Lief decided to arrange to have a series of treatments on himself from Varma, and finally persuaded the latter to teach him this specialized technique. Much as he appreciated the method used by Varma, he felt it could be improved, and began to develop and

subsequently practised the method for which he devised the name of 'Neuro-muscular Technique'. This name was an accurate definition of the purpose of the method he evolved from the rather crude technique used by Varma. This involved an application of hands and fingers to the appropriate areas of soft tissue related to the affected bony articulations, as well as all other areas of soft tissue which his sensitive fingers found to be abnormal in texture. This enables adverse factors in such tissue to be corrected to allow the full function of *muscles* and nerves to be re-established. In doing so the double benefits are achieved in improving nerve and blood circulation, improving texture of muscle tissue and in being better able to get effective results in manipulating the bony articulations involved, and assuring lasting integrity of their normal function.

Stanley Lief also maintained that bony joint lesions were not the only factors in the interference in nerve force integrity, but that tensions contractions, adhesions, muscle spasms and fibrositic contractures in soft tissues could in themselves constitute primary factors in disease causation by reducing effective nerve and blood circulation. To this end he developed his diagnostic sensitivity with his fingers so that in a few seconds of palpation over any area of the body, he was able to assess abnormalities present in relation to tensions, adhesions, spasms etc.

The body's integrity of prime health and its functional efficiency at a high level, depends not only on its chemistry influenced by the nature of the food and drink we ingest, but also on the effective nerve and blood circulation free of mechanical and functional obstructions. To this second vital purpose there is no formula devised by the osteopathic or chiropractic professions that will more effectively achieve the optimum result than the philosophy and technique devised by Stanley Lief. There is no single part of the body that he was not able to apply his method to to achieve remarkable physiological responses.

Stanley Lief's son, Peter, has described[27] the 'neuro-muscular' lesion as being associated with:

1. Congestion of the local connective tissues.
2. Disturbance of the acid-base balance of the connective tissues.
3. Fibrous infiltration (adhesions).
4. Chronic muscular contractions or hyper- or hypotrophic (tone) changes.

Etiology of the neuro-muscular lesion, according to Lief, include a number of causative factors, giving rise to neuro-muscular lesions, which may include:

1. Fatigue, exhaustion, bad posture.
2. Local trauma.
3. Systemic toxaemia (lack of exercise and oxygen).
4. Dietetic deficiencies.
5. Psychosomatic causes bringing about muscular tensions.

The presence of a lesion is always revealed by an area of hypersensitivity to pressure.

Tissues Involved in NMT

Boris Chaitow and Peter Lief have both evolved the theory and application of NMT as first described by Stanley Lief. Brian Youngs[28] has given the following general explanation of the tissues involved in NMT:

Site of Application
As the technique operates primarily on connective tissue it will be concentrated at those areas where such tissue is most dense, e.g. muscular origins and insertions, especially the broad aponeurotic insertions. The most frequent sites are the superior curved line of the occiput, the numerous insertions and origins of the large, medium and small muscles which attach to the vertebral column; the iliac-crest insertions; the intercostal insertions and abdominal-muscle insertions. Nevertheless, the technique can of course be applied to any area which requires it—head, face, wrists, etc. Connective tissue is, after all, ubiquitous.

To understand the therapeutic effect of the technique one must have some knowledge of the pathophysiology of the tissue upon which it operates. Connective tissue consists of a matrix containing cells and fibres. It was largely ignored until recently, but has now been made the subject of close study—and even international conferences—in regard to its structure and functions. Dr Rabagliatti, forty-five years ago, was so interested and far-seeing that his book, *Initis,* contained concepts the general truth of which is being proved today. He was, however, a lone voice and because he held unorthodox ideas he was, typically, ignored.

The ubiquity of connective tissue caused Dr Rabagliatti to analogize it to the ether—as the medium for, as he termed it, 'the zoodynamic life force'.

Through the connective tissues' planes run the trunks and plexuses of veins, arteries, nerves, and lymphatics. Connective tissue is the support for the structural and, therefore, functional relationships of these systems.

Chemical Structure
Briefly, the matrix consists of a jelly-like ground substance in which the fibres, cells, vessels, etc., lie. This ground substance is the 'physical expression of the *milieu intérieure* intervening everywhere between the blood and lymph vessels and the metabolizing cells; it plays a major role in the transport, storage and exchange of water and electrolytes. The chemical structure is essentially polysaccharide, hyaluronic acid, chondroitin sulphuric acid, chondroitin sulphate and chondroitin itself, together with proteins which contain a considerable amount of the amino acid tyrosine, which forms the majority of the thyroxin molecule.

The fibres are white fibrous (collagen), yellow (elastin), and reticulin. The collagen fibres are also protein and polysaccharide in composition and are stabilized chemically by the presence of the ground substance constituents. The presence of chondroitin sulphate, for example, renders the enzymatic breakdown of collagen much more difficult. The importance of this point will become more clear later. The formation of fibres appears to be due to a precipitation of fibre constituents by serum glycoproteins under the influence of adrenocorticotrophic hormone.

Reticulin contains more polysaccharide than collagen, and some lipid also. Elastin is also protein and polysaccharide in composition. Sulphur is a constituent of all three. Cells include fibroblasts, mast cells, macrophages and others.

A Function of Circulation
The nature and composition of connective tissue is a function of circulation. Circulatory efficiency in any area will determine (1) the influx of materials to the area, and (2) the drainage of the area.

Incoming blood leads to the production of lymph and this fluid permeates the ground substance, bringing all the constituents of the blood except the proteins to the connective tissue. Some of these constituents are hormones. Thyroxin, adrenogluco-corticoids and adrenomineralocorticoids are only three of these. Oestrogen and androgens are two more. All these have known effects upon the structure of connective tissue. Thus, a diminution of thyroxin leads to an increase of water retention in most cells and an increase in the quantity of ground substance. The sex hormones also do this, but of most interest to us, here are the opposing groups of the adrenocortical hormones. Selye divides these into anti- and pro-inflammatory hormones (A-Cs and P-Cs). These are produced in response to stress situations and they exert both a general and a local effect. By regulating the balance between these two the body can control the ability of the tissues to produce an inflammatory response. But when the A-Cs and the P-Cs are both present in the blood the A-Cs always win the contest, i.e., there is an anti-inflammatory response.

Stressor Stimulus

The A-Cs are produced in response to a stimulus—the stressor. The stressor in neuro-muscular technique is pain. Effective technique appears to be accompanied by pain in all (I generalize here deliberately) such conditions (and also in the condition without treatment). Pain is probably due to two factors. A much reduced threshold in the area due to circulatory inhibition enabling a build up to just below the threshold level of Lewis pain substance or, alternatively, a disturbance of electrolyte level (e.g., increase of hydrogen ions or disturbance in the calcium/sodium/potassium balance due to the same circumstances). Consequently pain will be produced by even slight stimulus, let alone the heavier movements of neuro-muscular technique. Also, pressure and tension proprioceptors may be overstimulated and pain can result from an over-application of any ordinary stimulus.

The A-Cs liberated will produce both general effects (General Adaptation Syndrome) and local effects (Local Adaptation Syndrome) and their effect is anti-inflammatory, both generally and locally, at the area of application of the stressor, i.e., at the areas of technique application. Consequently, there is a break-down of collagen fibres and a general decrease in water retention in the ground substance; the congested area is decongested.

We have now looked at the soft tissues through a variety of eyes. What emerges is the certainty that therapeutic effort is well aimed if directed at normalizing the neuro-muscular component (to include connective tissue) of any dysfunction. Whether the object is to improve local or general function or to prepare for active manipulation or to remove reflex pain patterns, the objects of attention are the soft-tissue structures with their altered feel and sensitivity to pressure. Various workers have described the same changes using different terminology and advising a variety of therapeutic methods. NMT offers a simple system of diagnosis and treatment based on over forty years of use and development. In skilled hands it can remove pain, improve function, obviate manipulation or prepare for it, enhance the body's economy, relieve stress, induce relaxation and well-being and greatly aid in the restoration of health—without side effects.

Before considering the technique itself it will be necessary to examine reflex symptoms and trigger areas which originate in the soft tissues.

[1] Erlinghauser, R. F., 'Circulation of C.S.F. Through Connective Tissues,' *Academy of Applied Osteopathy Yearbook* (1959).
[2] Selye, H., *The Stress of Life,* (McGraw Hill, 1956).
[3] Humphreys, P. W. and Lind, A. R., *Journal of Physiology* (1963), pp. 120-135.
[4] Jacobson, E., 'Principles Underlying Coronary Heart Disease,' *Cardiologia* (1955), pp. 26-83.
[5] Barlow, W., 'Anxiety and Muscle Tension Pain', *British Journal of Clinical Practice,* Vol. 3, No. 5.
[6] Alexander, F. M., *The Use of the Self,* (Educational Publications, 1957).

[7] Lewis, Sir Thomas, *Pain,* (New York, 1942).

[8] Reich, Wilhelm, *Character Analysis,* (Vision Press, 1949).

[9] Boadella, David, 'The Language of the Body in Bio-energetic Therapy', *Journal of the Research Society for Natural Therapeutics* (1978).

[10] Taylor, R. B., 'Bio-energetics of Man', *Academy of Applied Osteopathy Yearbook* (1958).

[11] Little, K. E., 'Toward More Effective Manipulative Management of Chronic Myofascial Strain and Stress Syndromes', *Journal of the American Osteopathic Association,* Vol. 68 (March, 1969).

[12] Eeman, L., *Co-operative Healing,* (Frederick Muller, 1947).

[13] Rolf, Ida, 'Structural Dynamics', *British Academy of Applied Osteopathy Yearbook* (1962).

[14] Taylor, R. B., *op. cit.*

[15] Gutstein, R., 'A Review of Myodysneuria (Fibrositis)', *American Practitioner and Digest of Treatments,* Vol. 6, No. 4.

[16] Petersen, W., *The Patient and the Weather: Autonomic Disintegration,* (Edward Bros., Ann Arbor, 1934).

[17] Bayer, H., Pathophysiology of Muscular Rheumatism., *Ztschr. Raeumaforsch 9:210 (1950)*

[18] Cathie, Dr A., 'Selected Writings', *Academy of Applied Osteopathy Yearbook* (1974).

[19] Pauling, Linus, *The Common Cold and 'Flu,* (W. H. Freeman and Company, 1976).

[20] Cyriax, J., *Textbook of Orthopaedic Medicine,* (Cassell, 1962).

[21] Stoddard, Dr Alan, *Manual of Osteopathic Practice,* (Hutchinson, 1969).

[22] Ebner, M., *Connective Tissue Massage,* (Churchill Livingstone, 1962).

[23] Lecture to Research Society for Natural Therapeutics, 1969.

[24] Korr, I., 'Spinal Cord as Organiser of Disease Process', *Academy of Applied Osteopathy Yearbook* (1976).

[25] Patterson, M., 'Model Mechanism for Spinal Segmental Facilitation', *Academy of Applied Osteopathy Yearbook* (1976).

[26] Personal communication to the author.

[27] Lief, P., *British Naturopathic Journal,* Vol. 5, No. 10.

[28] Youngs, B., 'Physiological Background of NM Technique', *British Naturopathic Journal,* Vol. 5, No. 6.

Chapter 2

Reflex Areas and
Somatic Dysfunction

Much work has been done in recent years in the field of myofascial trigger points. Janet Travell[1] M.D. has stated that if a pain is severe enough to cause a patient to seek professional advice it is usually a referred pain and therefore a trigger area is involved (if there is no evidence of organic or metabolic disease). She maintains that patterns of referred pain are constant in distribution in all people, only intensity will vary. Among the effects of an active trigger point there may be numbness, tingling, weakness, lack of normal range of movement as well as pain. The etiological myofascial trigger point for a particular pain pattern is always located in a particular part of a particular muscle.[2] Eradication of the trigger, by whatever means, will remove all symptoms. Treatment of the target or reference area is useless.

There is some disagreement about the role of bony or joint lesions in the maintenance of such pain patterns. One school of thought maintains that such 'lesions' should be corrected manipulatively, prior to dealing with the myofascial trigger. The importance of the fourth dorsal segment and the lumbo-dorsal junction is emphasized in this regard. Others, notably Travell, suggest such manipulative procedures should be performed after the myofascial pain pattern has been normalized.

Trigger Areas

The trigger areas, in so far as they concern our present study, are localized areas of deep tenderness and increased resistance. Pressure on such a trigger will often produce twitching and fasciculation. Pressure maintained on such a point will produce referred pain in a predictable area. If there are a number of active trigger points the reference areas may overlap. Any physical or psychic stress factor can result in alterations in normal tone in muscles, fascia and other soft tissues. This can affect changes in joint play, breathing, posture etc. and result in abnormal and constant tension. This in turn can lead to swelling, myositis and spasm which is the predisposing condition in the production of trigger points and their referred pain and dysfunction. Trauma or chilling may also be part of the etiology.

A number of methods exist for the obliteration of such trigger points, ranging from pharmacological agents such as novocaine or xylocain, to coolant sprays and acupuncture techniques. It is noteworthy that direct pressure techniques can also effectively reduce and ultimately remove such trigger areas. In so far as such a course of action would fit into neuro-muscular treatment it is of value to this study. Individual preference for one or other technique will allow scope for the effective removal of these pain sources. It is important to remember that a trigger point is self-perpetuating unless it is correctly treated.

Once symptoms have been relieved the muscle containing the trigger must be gently stretched to its longest resting length. Failing this, symptoms will return, irrespective of the technique used (chilling, pressure, injection, acupuncture etc.). Such stretching should be gradual and gentle.

Dr J. Mennell[3] states that a muscle that can attain and maintain its normal resting length is a pain-free muscle. One that cannot (a muscle in spasm) is usually a source of pain, regardless of whether the source of the spasm is in that muscle or not. Whatever the means used to 'block' the trigger activity and whatever the neuropathological routes involved, the critical factor in the restoration of pain-free normality is that during any relief from the state of spasm or contraction, the affected muscle should have its normal resting length restored by stretching. Mennell defines trigger points as localized palpable spots of deep hypersensitivity from which noxious impulses bombard the CNS to give rise to referred pain. Mennell favours chilling the trigger area by vapo-coolant or ice-massage. Details of his recommended method will be given in the treatment section.

Gutstein   There are many factors involved in the role of reflexes in both pathological and physiological activity. Neuro-muscular Technique provides the opportunity to both seek out reflex trigger areas and to treat them manually. It further allows for the application of other reflex effects. Gutstein[4] has shown that conditions such as ametropia may result from changes in the neuro-muscular component of the craniocervical area as well as more distant conditions involving the pelvis or shoulder girdle. He states:

> Myopia is the long-term effect of pressure of extraocular muscles in the convergence effort of accommodation and by spasm of the ciliary muscles, with resultant elongation of the eyeball. A sequential relationship has been shown between such a condition and muscular spasm of the neck.

Normalization of these muscles by manipulation relieves eye symptoms as well as fascial, dorsolumbar and abdominal tenderness. Gutstein terms these reflexes 'myodysneuria' and suggests that the reference phenomena of such spots or triggers would include pain, modifications of pain, itching, hypersensitivity to physiological stimuli, spasm, twitching, weakness and trembling of striated muscles; hyper- or hypo-tonus of smooth muscle of blood vessels, and of internal organs; hyper- or hypo-secretion of visceral, sebaceous and sudatory glands. Somatic manifestations may also occur in response to visceral stimuli of corresponding spinal levels.

Many such trigger areas are dormant and asymptomatic. Gutstein's method of treatment is the injection of an anaesthetic solution into the trigger area. He indicates however that where accessible (e.g. muscular insertions in the cervical area) the chilling of these areas combined with pressure will yield good results. This is in line with Mennell's work and fits into the field of Neuro-muscular Technique. Amongst the patterns of vasomotor sebaceous, sudatory and gastro-intestinal dysfunction quoted by Gutstein are the following, all of which relate to reflex trigger points or 'myodysneuria'.

1. Various patterns of vasomotor abnormality such as coldness, pallor, redness, cyanosis etc. The variations in response to stimulation relates to the fact that most organs respond to weak stimuli by an increase in activity and to very strong stimuli by inhibiting activity. Menopausal hot flushes are one example and these seem often to be linked with musculoskeletal pain. Gutstein found that obliteration of overt and silent triggers in the occipital, cervical, interscapular, sternal and epigastric regions was accompanied by years of alleviation of premenopausal, menopausal and late menopausal symptoms. NMT has long emphasized the importance of normalizing these very structures.

2. Gutstein maintains that normalization of skin secretion and therefore of hair and skin texture and appearance may be altered for the better by the removal of active trigger areas in the cervical and interscapular areas.

3. The conditions of hyper- and hypo- and an-hidrosis accompany vasomotor and sebaceous dysfunction. The trigger areas were similar and it was often found that abolition of excessive perspiration as well as anhidrosis followed adequate treatment.

4. Gutstein quotes a number of practitioners who have achieved success in treating gastro-intestinal dysfunctions by treating trigger areas. Some of these were treated by procainization, others by pressure techniques and massage. The abdominal wall lends itself to this latter procedure as evidenced by the work of Cornelius[5] whose treatment was not dissimilar to that of Lief's NMT.

Among the conditions that have responded to such treatment are the following:

Pylorospasm, bad breadth, heartburn, regurgitation, nausea, abdominal distension, constipation, nervous diarrhoea etc.

Obviously other causes, notably of a dietary nature, might be involved. However, in a number of instances the 'trigger' points might well be the major factor.

The main area of these triggers, relating to gastro-intestinal dysfunction, were found to be in the upper, mid and lower portions of the rectus muscles, over the lower portion of the sternum, the epigastrium, including the xiphoid process and the parasternal regions. The latter correspond with the insertions of the three portions of the rectus muscle into the cartilages of the fifth, sixth and seventh ribs. These triggers are found by careful palpation and pressure *(see illustration on page 108)*.

Travell and Bigelow[6] have produced evidence that supports much of what Gutstein has reported. They indicate that high intensity stimuli from active trigger areas produce, by reflex, prolonged vaso-constriction with partial ischaemia in localized areas of the brain, spinal cord, or peripheral nerve structures. There might result a wide pattern of dysfunction affecting almost any organ of the body. The phenomenon of hysteria with symptoms as varied as disordered vision, respiration, motor power and cutaneous sensation, were often mediated by afferent neural impulses from trigger areas in skeletal muscle. These triggers when similarly located, produced the same pattern of clinical effects, whether activated in one patient by psychogenic factors or in another by other factors (e.g. mechanical or traumatic).

Reflex Pain   Evans[7] in discussing reflex pain describes the mechanism as follows:

> A prolonged bombardment of pain impulses sets up a vicious circle of reflexes spreading through a pool of many neuron connections upward, downward and even across the spinal cord and perhaps reaching as high as the thalamus itself. Depending upon the extent of the pool (internuncial pool), we detect the phenomena of pain and sympathetic disturbances a long distance from the injured (trigger) area of the body and occasionally even spread to the contra-lateral side.

Dittrich[8] has shown a constant pattern of fibrosis of subfascial tissue, with adhesions between this and the overlying muscle fascia, in a number of distinctive and common pain patterns. In what he calls the 'mid-sacral syndrome' which develops from sacral lesions, referred pain is almost always present in the buttock and sometimes in the thigh, leg or foot. Referred tenderness is elicited in the lower part of the buttock. The fibrous adhesions (trigger area) are found at the level of the *third sacral vertebra near the spine.*

In the 'mid-lumbar syndrome' there is referred pain and tenderness in the lower lumbar, upper sacral and sacro-iliac regions. The trigger point is found over the lateral third of the sacro-spinalis muscle at the level of the *upper margin of the iliac crest.*

The 'latissimus-dorsi syndrome' may result from irritation of the *aponeurosis of this muscle* at either of the sites of injury, sacral or lumbar mentioned above. Referred pain would develop in the sclerotonic distributions of the sixth, seventh, and eighth cervical nerves.

He points out that pathological changes at the two sites have been discovered by operative findings. His technique is to surgically remove these triggers or to obliterate the triggers by injection of local anaesthetic. No concern is expressed for the mechanical, postural or other reasons that may have produced them, nor is any mention made of more conservative manipulative methods of normalization. The presence of 'fibrosed subfascial tissue' supports the theories of Stanley Lief and Boris Chaitow. The locale of these, close to bony insertions, further supports the rationale behind Neuro-muscular Technique.

It seems that soft tissue lesions, characterized by fibrosis of subfascial tissue (fat etc.) with fibrous connections between the structure and the overlying fascia can initiate sensory irritation which produce referred pain and tenderness. In addition, autonomic nervous involvement may be activated to produce vaso-motor, trophic, viseral or metabolic changes. Symptoms will disappear when the offending lesion is normalized by whatever method. However, a system that both corrects the offending trigger and attempts to prevent its recurrence would seem to have a greater scientific basis.

M. Blashey M.D.[9], dealing with limb rehabilitation, describes the research of **Fuchs' System**
Julius Fuchs, a Germany orthopaedist who died in 1953. Fuchs' system used
supporting structures of a part elastic material and part non-elastic material
which was arranged so that antagonistic muscle groups were supported in such a
way as to produce 'kinetic fields'. These fields were kinetically facilitating where
elastic tissue was used and kinetically impeding where inelastic tissue was used.
However, where sensory nerve damage had occurred in the skin overlying these
muscles no kinetic effect was obtained. Only light pressure on the muscular
structures involved was found to be required to produce what Fuchs termed the
'orthokinetic' effect.

From this research we learn a good deal about the reflex effect on muscle
groups that light manipulation of the overlying tissue of affected muscles can
produce. Does there exist a specific function of structure or both, connecting
skin surface with underlying muscle, in a direct and specific manner? It would
seem so.

Hagbarth[10] has shown that both flexor and extensor responses can be elicited
in a definite structural pattern. In the knee, for example, the flexors can be
stimulated from the skin of the entire limb *apart* from the skin overlying the
extensors. (In his experiments he was using the cat as a model but later work has
shown it to be valid for humans). The skin overlying the extensors is exitatory for
the extensors. The converse applies, so that all skin covering the flexors is
inhibitory for the extensors. This is summarized below:

Table 1. Areas of Inhibition and Excitation with Flexor and Extensor Responses in the Knee

Motion of Knee	Area of Inhibition	Area of Excitation
Flexion	over extensors only	over rest of limb
Extension	over flexors only	over rest of limb

These effects were obtained thermally, electrically and by tactile stimulation
which did not need to be heavy. The 'skin motor areas' or 'orthokinetic fields'
do not correspond in distribution to the skin fields of cutaneous nerves or with
segmental arrangements.

I do not intend to become involved in the theoretical hypothetical neurological arguments that support these clinical facts. For the purposes of the study
of neuro-muscular treatment the existence of a particular effect is in itself
adequate. Physiologists, anatomists, biologists and zoologists will eventually
produce profound definitive answers to all such conundrums. In the mean time,
as in the case of acupuncture, the ethical practitioner can use knowledge gained
by clinical means with equanimity as long as it is demonstrated that no harm can
stem from the procedures involved. Such is the case in the present example.

To summarize this finding: there is a definite functional connection between a
muscle and the portion of skin that covers it. They are integrated so that muscle
is excited by stimuli within its own skin area. This area will be inhibitory to the
antagonist of the underlying muscle.

Connective Tissue Massage

A system which incorporates a great deal of reflex effects is connective tissue massage (CTM). CTM involves the use of 'rolling' the tissues in order to achieve reflex and local effects. The strokes pull and stretch the tissues and it is suggested[11] that its effectiveness is based on a viscerocutaneous reflex. Bischof and Elmiger explain it thus:

> The specific mechanical stimulation of the pull on connective tissue seems to be the adequate stimulus to elicit the nervous reflex. Connective tissue massage acts first on the sympathetic terminal reticulum in the skin. The smallest branches of the autonomic nervous system contact the impulses activated by the pulling strokes to the sympathetic trunk and the spinal cord. The impulses travel from the skin either through a somatosensory spinal nerve via a posterior root ganglion to the grey matter or over the vascular plexus to the same segmental sympathetic ganglion or to the ganglion of the neighbouring segment, through the ramus communicans albus to the posterior root and grey matter of the spinal cord. They terminate either directly or by means of the internuncial neurons at the efferent autonomic root cells.
>
> In the efferent pathway the impulses travel from the autonomic lateral horn, or the intermediolateral column, over the anterior root, ramus communicans albus, to the segmental sympathetic ganglion or to the ganglion of the neighbouring segment and finally to the diseased organ. The origin of the connective tissue reflex zones and the influence of the CTM depend on the relationship between the function of the internal organs, vessels, and nerves as well as the tissues of the locomotor apparatus, which descend from the same metamere.

> Clara reminds us that the human embryo is composed of many homogeneous primitive segments (metameres) that are arranged serially. This arrangement is concerned with the mesoderm and the tissue regions derived from it—sclerotomes, myotomes, dermatomes, (ectoderm), angiotomes and nephrotomes. Secondly, the ectoderm participates in the segmentation (metamerism) since in each of the primitive segments or metameres one corresponding spinal nerve enters. The skin over the segment is also innervated, and in this way the segmentation is projected to the skin. This embryonal connection between the primitive segment and the spinal nerve (dermatome) develops early and remains unchanged postembryonically. Head was the first to point out that the internal organs that develop from the entoderm correspond to certain spinal cord segments, although the entoderm does not participate in the segmentation. The relationship between tissues and their spinal root innervation is the scientific foundation for CTM and other forms of segmental therapy. Most investigators differ little in their reports concerning the segmental connections of the internal organs. Different schemes have been proposed by Hansen, Keegan, Dejerine and others to relate skin topography with the internal organs.

During and after Connective Tissue Massage there are a number of reflex reactions including vaso-dilatation and diffuse or localized sweating. Some of these reflexes do not seem to be segmental in nature. For example, dilatation of the upper extremity blood vessels occurs when the pelvis is treated by CTM. The maximal skin temperature increase occurs about half an hour after CTM is discontinued and persists for an hour or so. It is of interest that the vaso-dilatory effect of CTM is as pronounced, or even more pronounced, after lumbar sympathectomy.

Some of the reactions to CTM are normal autonomic responses such as pleasant fatigue, bowel movements and diuresis. Oedema is markedly reduced and hormonal distribution is seen to achieve a degree of balance. Aspects of

CTM are similar to NMT, and the 'skin rolling' methods used in some body areas are virtually identical in application. The effects are therefore interesting from a comparative point of view.

A further reflex pattern has been described by Chapman and Owens. In an earlier work[12] I described these as follows:

Chapman's Reflexes

> The reflexes of Chapman that I intend to discuss now are not the whole picture—they are only a part of the visible portion of the iceberg—but of immense value nonetheless.
>
> Drs Chapman and Owens first reported on Chapman's original findings in the late 1930s. A revised edition of their work has recently been published by the Academy of Applied Osteopathy.
>
> The surface changes of a Chapman's Reflex are palpable. They may best be described as contractions located in specific anatomical areas and always associated with the same viscera. In describing each organ reflex Chapman normally indicated tissue reflex areas, occurring anteriorly and posteriorly. These reflexes found in the deep fascia are described as 'gangliform' contractions. These contractions vary in size from a pellet to a large bean and are located anteriorly in the intercostal spaces near the sternum. Similar tissue changes are found in those reflexes occurring on the pelvis. The tissue changes found in reflexes located on the lower extremeties are described as 'stringy masses' or 'amorphous shotty plaques'. Those reflexes occurring posteriorly along the spine, midway between the spinal processes and the tips of the transverse processes are of a more oedematous nature.
>
> *The Value of the Reflexes*
> Since the location of these palpable tissue changes is constant in relation to specific viscera it is possible to establish the location of pathology without knowing its nature. The value of these reflexes is threefold:
> 1. As diagnostic aids.
> 2. They can be utilized to influence the motion of fluids, mostly lymph.
> 3. Visceral function can be influenced through the nervous system.
>
> *The Mechanism of the Reflexes*
> As to the mechanism whereby these reflexes act, it would appear that, in so far as the intercostal reflexes are concerned, stimulation of the receptor organs which lie between the anterior and posterior layers of anterior intercostal fascia acts through the intercostal nerve which enervates the external and internal intercostal muscles and thus, through the sympathetic fibres, affects the intercostal arteries, veins, lymph nodes, etc. Stimulation thus causes afferent and efferent vessels draining these tissues to increase or decrease, permitting lymph flow to be increased or decreased thus affecting the drainage of the entire lymph system in the area. Through the sympathetic fibres associated with these tissues the lymph nodes of the vital organs are also affected.
>
> *Explaining Results of Neuro-muscular Technique*
> In my own mind I have no doubt that a knowledge of these reflexes goes a good way to explaining the sometimes startling results obtained through Neuro-muscular Technique. Stanley Lief placed great emphasis on the intercostal spaces and the paravertebral areas; he also stressed the importance of not over-treating, a consideration which cannot be repeated too often.

Reference to these reflexes will be found in the chapter on treatment techniques.

The soft tissues are of major importance to the body's economy, structural integrity and well being. They are also a major source of pain and dysfunction and, as must now be obvious, of reflex disturbances.

Acupuncture Points
Soft tissue changes often produce organized discrete areas which act as generators of secondary problems, it would be advantageous to examine briefly another aspect of 'trigger' points, that is, the existence of a network of points which is supposedly constantly capable of reflex activity. This network is, of course, the pattern of acupuncture points. What is of interest is that the location of these fixed anatomical points is capable of corroboration by electrical detection, each point being evidenced by a small area of lowered electrical resistance.

When 'active', due presumably to reflex, stimulation of some kind these points become even more detectable, as the electrical resistance lowers further. They also become sensitive to pressure and this is of value to the therapist since the finding of sensitive areas during palpation or treatment is of diagnostic interest. Sensitive and painful areas that do not have detectable tissue changes as part of their make-up may well be 'active' acupuncture points (or *Tsubo,* which means 'points on the human body' in Japanese). Not only are these points detectable and sensitive but are also amenable to treatment by direct pressure techniques. They are, therefore, well worth some study.

One of the leading oriental experts on pressure techniques is Katsusuke Serizawe M.D. who, in his book on the subject, discusses his nerve-reflex theory for the existence of these points.

The nerve reflex theory holds that, when an abnormal condition occurs in an internal organ, alterations take place in the skin and muscles related to that organ by means of the nervous system. These alterations occur as reflex actions. The nervous system, extending throughout the internal organs, like the skin, the subcutaneous tissues, and the muscles, constantly transmit information about the physical condition to the spinal cord and the brain. These information impulses, which are centripetal in nature, set up a reflex action that causes symptoms of the internal organic disorder to manifest themselves in the surface areas of the body. The reflex symptoms may be classified into the following three major groups: (a) sensation reflexes; (b) interlocking reflexes; (c) autonomic system reflexes.

(a) Sensation reflexes. When an abnormal centripetal impulse travels to the spinal cord, reflex action causes the skin at the spinal column affected by the impulse to become hypersensitive. This sensitivity to pain is especially notable in the skin, subcutaneous tissues, and muscles located close to the surface, since these organs are richly supplied with sensory nerves.

(b) Interlocked reflexes. An abnormality in an internal organ causes a limited contraction, stiffening, or lumping of the muscles in the area near the part of the body that is connected by means of nerves to the affected organ. Stiffness in the shoulders, back, arms, and legs are symptoms of this kind. In effect, the interlocked reflex actions amount to a hardening and stiffening of the muscles to protect the ailing internal organ from excess stimulus. When the abnormality in the organ is grave, however, the stiffening of the muscles is not limited to a small area, but extends over large parts of the body.

(c) Autonomic system reflexes. Abnormalities in the internal organs sometimes set up reflex action in the sweat glands, the sebaceous glands, the pilomotor muscles, and the blood vessels in the skin. The reflex action may cause excess sweat or drying of the skin as the consequence of cessation of sweat secretion. Its effect on the pilomotor muscles may be to cause the condition known as goose flesh. The sebaceous glands may be stimulated to secrete excess sebum, thus causing abnormal oiliness in the skin; or they may stop secreting sebum, thus making the skin abnormally dry. The reflex action may cause chills or flushing because of its effects on the blood vessels in the skin.

I have discussed the ways in which abnormalities in internal organs cause changes in the conditions of the surface organs of the body. But the intimate relation between internal organs and external ones has a reverse effect as well; that is, stimulation to the skin and muscles affects the condition of the internal organs and tissues, since impulses from the outside are transmitted to the inside by means of the spinal cord and the nervous system. For instance, stimulation transmitted to the spinal cord sets up a reflex action in the internal organ that is controlled by the nerves at the level of the spinal column corresponding to the height of the place at which the external stimulus was applied. Stimuli of this kind instigate peristaltic motion or contraction in the organ. The effect of such external stimulation on blood vessels and on the secretion of hormones has been scientifically verified.

Quite obviously there may be more effective ways of dealing with these points than by pressure techniques. However, since the study is concerned basically with manual treatment it is worth incorporating into our scheme of treatment the knowledge accumulated by the Chinese and Japanese over many centuries.

An attempt to correlate the various reflex systems and methods has been made by the American Chiropractor Dr George Goodheart. His system of Applied Kinesiology involves testing muscle groups for weaknesses and then, depending upon the results of such tests, using various massage and pressure techniques in order to normalize function. These points correspond to Chapman's reflexes, acupuncture points and other less well known reflex systems. It is not my intention to delve into Goodheart's techniques and theories, some of which seem far-fetched to a practical observer—he claims that muscles can be strengthened by passing a hand along the line of the 'energy' flow of an acupuncture meridian, without even touching the patient. However, where his methods support and utilize methods that are in line with Neuro-muscular Technique these will be mentioned in the treatment section.

It has been shown that the pain threshold can be dramatically elevated by pressure techniques on specific points. In complex experiments the research group of acupuncture anaesthesia, Peking Medical College, showed that finger pressure acupuncture caused a rise of 133 per cent in pain threshold of rabbits (using radiant heat as the painful stimulus). When cerebrospinal fluid was perfused from one rabbit to another after such experiments the recipient rabbit was found to have achieved a rise in pain threshold of up to 80 per cent. This suggests the presence of hormone-like substances produced by the brain in response to the original acupressure stimulus. These substances, now thought to be enkephalin and endorphin, may well play a role in NMT pain control. The point used in these tests was equivalent to the acupuncture point known as Bladder 60, posterior to the ankle (externally) and just anterior to the Achilles tendon.

The various theories, methods and descriptive terminologies relating to the foregoing systems are of some general interest in as much as Neuro-muscular Technique overlaps and incorporates many aspects that are similar. This should not be confusing as there are many ways of looking at the same phenomena.

Neuro-muscular Technique can (with other modalities such as chilling agents) be used as an effective measure to detect and eliminate noxious trigger points and areas which generate dysfunction. Such dysfunction can take the form of muscular weakness, muscular contraction, pain, vaso-dilatation, vaso-constriction, tissue degeneration, gastro-intestinal, respiratory and a myriad other disorders including emotional and 'psychological' disorders.

These noxious points may reside in hypertonic or hypotonic muscle or in ligamentous or fascial tissues, or in apparently normal tissues. When active, they will always be sensitive to correctly applied pressure and can often be neutralized by manual pressure or a combination of chilling and manual pressure and stretching.

We now know what these triggers are, and the types of problems they can cause. In the treatment section we will discuss how to locate and treat them.

[1] Travell, Dr J., 'Symposium on Mechanism and Management of Pain Syndromes', *Proc. Rudolph Virchow Medical Soc.* (1957).

[2] Webber, T. D., 'Diagnosis and Modification of Headache and Shoulder, Arm, Hand Syndromes', *Journal of the American Osteopathic Association,* Vol. 72 (March, 1973).

[3] Mennell, Dr J., 'The Therapeutic Use of Cold', *Journal of the American Osteopathic Association,* Vol. 74 (August, 1975).

[4] Gutstein, R., 'The Role of Craniocervical Myodysneuria in Functional Ocular Disorders', *American Practitioner's Digest of Treatments* (November, 1956).

[5] Cornelius, A., *Die Neurenpunkt Lehre Vol. 2* (George Thins, Liepzig).

[6] Travell, J. and Bigelow, N., 'Role of Somatic Trigger Areas in the Patterns of Hysteria', *Psychosomatic Medicine,* Vol. 9, No. 6.

[7] Evans, J., 'Reflex Sympathetic Dystrophy', *Annals of Internal Medicine*

[8] Dittrich, R. J., 'Somatic Pain and Autonomic Concomitants', *American Journal of Surgery* (1954).

[9] Blashy, M., 'Manipulation of the Neuromuscular Unit via the Periphery of the CNS', *Southern Medical Journal* (August, 1961).

[10] Hagbarth, K., 'Excitatory Inhibitory Skin Areas for Flexor and Extensor Motoneurons', *Acta Physiologica Scandinavia* (1952).

[11] Bischof, I. and Elmiger, G., 'Connective Tissue Massage', *Massage, Manipulation and Traction* (Licht, 1960).

[12] Chaitow, Leon, 'An Introduction to Chapman's Reflexes', *British Naturopathic Journal* (Spring, 1965).

Chapter 3

Diagnostic Methods

In the previous chapters we have dipped into the vast amount of information that exists relating to the neuro-muscular component of the human framework. An equally great number of diagnostic aids exist for the researcher into the ills of the body. The great beauty of Neuro-muscular Technique, as devised by Lief, is its combining of diagnostic and therapeutic movements. The thumb as it glides close to the spinal attachments of the paraspinal musculature is assessing the tissue tone, density, temperature etc., and at the same moment is treating those tissues that indicate dysfunction, by means of variable pressure. The response of the searching digit to whatever information the tissues impart, is immediate. Greater or lesser pressure, varying in its direction and duration, allows the practitioner to judge and treat at the same time and with great accuracy.

In a general sense, on a level involving the whole of an area or the total body picture, a diagnostic or assessment plan is required. Whilst the individual muscular indurations and dysfunctions will become apparent as treatment progresses, an overall diagnostic picture is required to enable prognosis and progress to be judged.

There is no valid substitute for skilful palpatory diagnosis in ascertaining the relatively minute structural changes—primary or reflex—that often have far-reaching effects on the body's economy.

It is generally agreed that the pads of the figures are the most sensitive portion of the hand available for use in diagnosis. Indeed the combination of the thumb and first two fingers is the finest mechanism, and can be adapted to vary with the area under palpatory consideration as to the practitioner's own preference.

Palpatory Diagnosis

The most successful method of palpatory diagnosis is to run lightly over the area being checked, seeking changes in the skin and the tissues below it. After localizing any changes in this way, deeper periaxial structures can be assessed by greater pressure. There are a number of specific changes to be sought in light palpatory examination. This applies to both acute and chronic dysfunction. Among these are:

1. *Skin changes.* Over an area of acute dysfunction, skin will feel tense and will be relatively difficult to move or glide over the underlying structures.

2. *Induration.* A slight increase in diagnostic pressure will ascertain whether or not the superficial musculature has an increased indurated feeling. When chronic dysfunction exists the skin and superficial musculature will demonstrate a tension and immobility indicating fibrotic changes within and below these structures.

3. *Temperature changes.* In acute dysfunction a localized increase in temperature may be evident. In chronic lesion conditions there may, because of relative ischaemia, be a reduced temperature of the skin. This usually indicates fibrotic alterations in the underlying structures.

4. *Tenderness.* Tenderness can be misleading as it may indicate local or reflex problems in acute or chronic dysfunction. Its presence should be noted but not necessarily considered to be important. In acute joint dysfunction the superficial musculature and skin usually palpates as tender.

5. *Oedema.* An impression of fullness and congestion can be obtained in the overlying tissues in acute dysfunction. In chronic dysfunction this is usually absent having been replaced by fibrotic changes.

In deep palpation the pressure of the palpating fingers or thumb increases sufficiently to make contact with deeper structures such as the periaxial (paravertebral) musculature. Amongst the changes noted may be immobility, tenderness, oedema, deep muscle tension, fibrotic and interosseous changes. Apart from the fibrotic changes, which are indicative of chronic dysfunctions, all these changes can be found in either acute or chronic problems.

As Peter Lief D.O., son of the innovator of Neuro-muscular Technique, explains:

Palpation is the main method of detection. Gross lesions are easily palpable but sometimes they are so minute that their detection presents considerable difficulty, especially to the beginner. It sometimes takes many months of practice to develop the necessary sense of touch, which must be firm, yet at the same time sufficiently light, in order to discern the minute tissue changes which constitute the palpable neuro-muscular lesion.

The presence of a lesion is always revealed by an area of hyper-sensitivity to pressure, an area which may be better described as being a painful spot. After these have been detected and noted, specific attention is given to them in the subsequent treatments.

Brian Youngs D.O. has described what it is that the palpating fingers are seeking and finding and, since in NMT diagnosis and treatment often take place together, what they are achieving.

The changes which are palpable in muscles and soft tissues associated with such reflex effects have been listed by Stanley Lief. They are essentially 'congestion'. This ambiguous word can be interpreted as a past hypertrophic fibrosis. Reflex cordant contraction of the muscle reduces the blood flow through the muscular tissue and in such relatively anoxic regions of low pH and low hormonal concentration, fibroblasts proliferate and increased fibrous tissue is formed. This results in an increase in the thickness of the existing connective tissue partitions—the epimysia and perimysia—and also this condition probably infiltrates deeper between the muscle fibres to affect the normal endomysia. Thickening of the fascia and subdermal connective tissue will also occur if these structures are similarly affected by a reduced blood flow. Fat may be deposited, particularly in endomorphic types, but fibrosis is most pronounced in those with a strong mesomorphic component—a useful pointer for both prognosis and prophylaxis.

Fibrosis seems to occur automatically in areas of reduced blood flow, e.g., in a sprained ankle—where swelling is marked and prolonged, in the lower extremities where oedema of any origin has been constant over a period, in the gluteals where prolonged sitting is a postural factor, and in the neck and upper dorsal region where psychosomatic tension is frequent to a marked degree—depending upon the constitutional background. Where tension is the etiological factor, fibrosis seems teleological. Many devices have been developed to ease the strain on muscles which tend to be permanently contracted, e.g., locking of the knee joint, or the exact balance of the head on the shoulders, where only gentle contraction is needed to maintain postural integrity. If postural integrity is lost through some cause or another then the strain on the muscle may be eased by structural alteration and the increase of fibrous tissue in the muscles acts to maintain normal position of the head. Fibrous tissue can then take the strain instead of the muscle fibres. It is this long-term homeostatic reflex which apparently operates in all cases of undue muscle contraction, whether due to strain or tension.

From this one can amplify Mr Lief's beneficial effects of neuro-muscular treatment as follows:

1. To restore muscular balance and tone.

2. To restore normal trophicity in muscular and connective tissues by altering the histological picture from a patho-histological to a physiologic-histological pattern with normal vascular and hormonal response.

3. To affect reflexly the related organs and viscera and to tonify them naturally.

4. To improve drainage of blood and lymph through the areas subject to gravitational or postural stasis, e.g., abdominal vessels not necessarily connected with viscera.

5. To reduce fatty deposits.

Thus the hyperaemia resulting from treatment automatically operates to reverse the original patho-histological picture and consequently normality will be approached.

The position of the practitioner and the patient and the various body structures, areas and tissues will be discussed in a later chapter. Apart from the tissue changes as mentioned above there should be an awareness of the reflex pathways and activities affecting and affected by each area being worked on. In this way the hands of the operator will yield a great fund of knowledge of the body which they are working on, as well as directly and reflexly aiding the achievement of homeostatic equilibrium.

In seeking the cause of pain and other symptoms knowledge of the patterns of reflex activity and 'target areas' is obviously a useful diagnostic aid. There is clinical evidence that trigger points have a consistent localization and their localization can be predicted by studying the patterns of referred dysfunction and pain to which they give rise. These patterns of referred pain are, of course, predictable if the trigger point is found. Thus the point at which the patient feels pain and the point at which the pain originates are often not the same. This emphasizes the importance of accurate palpation in physical examination. Whether treatment is going to consist of anaesthetic injections, acupuncture, cryotherapy or pressure and stretch techniques (NMT) the diagnostic aspect remains the same. Deep palpation and pressure must reproduce the symptoms in the target area by irritating the trigger point.

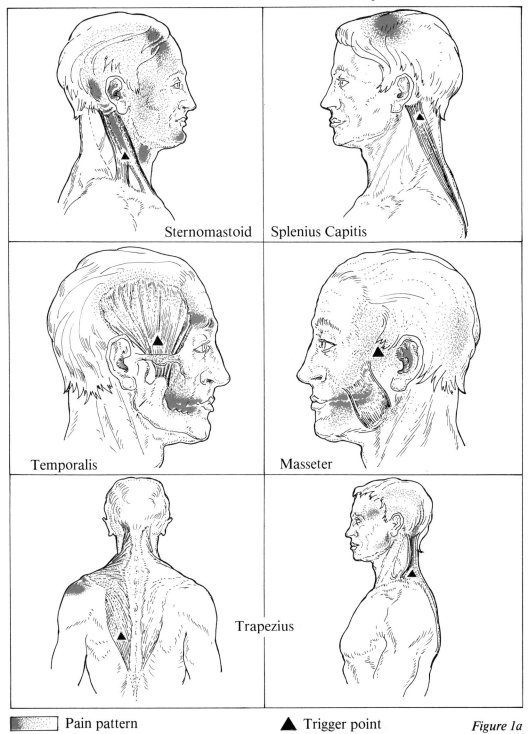

Sternomastoid   Splenius Capitis

Temporalis   Masseter

Trapezius

▨ Pain pattern   ▲ Trigger point

Figure 1a

Myofascial trigger points and usual areas of referred pain.

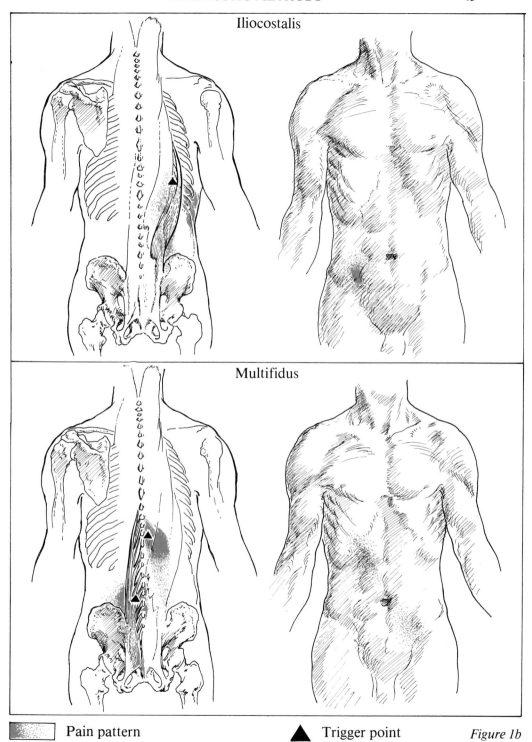

Pain pattern ▲ Trigger point

Figure 1b

Myofascial trigger points and usual areas of referred pain.

Levator Scapulae

Posterior Cervical

Infraspinatus

Supraspinatus

Adductor Pollicis

Pain pattern ▲ Trigger point

Figure 1c

Myofascial trigger points and usual areas of referred pain.

Scaleni

Deltoid

Subscapularis

First Interosseus

Pain pattern ▲ Trigger point *Figure 1d*

Myofascial trigger points and usual areas of referred pain.

Extensor Carpi Radialis

Supinators

Middle Finger Extensor

Pectoralis Major

Pectorals

Serratus Anterior

Pain pattern ▲ Trigger point

Figure 1e

Myofascial trigger points and usual areas of referred pain.

Gluteus Medius

Iliocostalis

Sternalis

Longissimus

Gastrocnemius

Soleus

Abductor Hallucis

Pain pattern   ▲ Trigger point   *Figure 1f*

Myofascial trigger points and usual areas of referred pain.

Tibialis Anticus

Gluteus Minimus

Long Extensors

Biceps Femoris

Short Extensors

Adductor Longus

Vastus Medialis

Peroneus Longus

▨ Pain pattern   ▲ Trigger point   *Figure 1g*

Myofascial trigger points and usual areas of referred pain.

Dr Janet Travell was the main charter of these points and their target areas. As well as the trigger points discussed above there exist a number of palpable and often visible zones of altered soft tissue resulting from disturbed organs and functions. These areas lend themselves to neuro-muscular treatment, especially Lief's basic spinal treatment (to be discussed later). Some of these zones overlap and incorporate 'trigger' points. A general awareness and knowledge of their existence is certainly vital to an adequate understanding of what is being achieved in treatment. Since organs mainly receive their autonomic supply homolaterally, changes of a reflex nature will normally be found on the same side of the body surface. On the right side will be found the reflex zones from the liver, gall bladder, duodenum, appendix, ascending colon and ilium etc.

On the left side will be found the reflex zones from the heart, stomach, pancreas, spleen, jejunum, transverse colon, descending colon and rectum etc. Central zones occur as a result of dysfunction in the bladder, uterus and the head. Changes on the corresponding side of the body occur due to dysfunction of the lungs, suprarenal glands, ovaries, kidneys, blood vessels and nerves. According to Ebner[1] these changes in the connective tissue and muscles can take any of the following forms, drawn in bands of tissues, flattened areas of tissue, elevated areas, giving the impression of localized swelling; muscle atrophy or hypertrophy; osseous deformity of the spinal column.

Teiriche-Leube[2] and Ebner describe some of these zones in the following terms:

Table 2. Altered Soft Tissue Zones Resulting from Disturbed Organs and Functions, Giving Location and Symptoms

Illustration	Zone	Location	Symptoms
1	Bladder	Small, 'drawn in' area above anal cleft. Iliotibial tract may be drawn in. Swelling lateral aspect of ankles.	Bladder dysfunction. Cold feet and legs (below the knee). Rheumatic diagnosis.
2	Constipation	'Drawn in' band 2 to 3 inches (5-8cm) wide running from middle third of the sacrum downwards and laterally.	Tendency to or actual constipation.
3	Liver and gall bladder	Large 'drawn in' zone over right thoracic region and a band along lateral costal border on the right side. Small 'drawn in' area between lower vertebral border of scapula to spine at the fifth and sixth dorsal level. Seventh cervical area appears swollen or congested.	Liver and gall bladder dysfunction and anyone who has suffered from hepatitis.

Illustration	Zone	Location	Symptoms
4	Heart	Tension over left thoracic region including lower costal margin. If hepatic circulation is involved right costal margin will also be affected. The area between the left scapula and second and third dorsal vertebrae will be indurated. Posterior aspect of axilla appears thickened.	Coronary and valvular diseases of the heart.
5	Stomach	Overlapping the heart zones (above). Localized tension area below lateral aspect of the left scapular spine.	Stomach dysfunction. Gastric ulcer and gastritis.
6	Arterial disease of legs	A V-shaped configuration of the buttocks when sitting is noticed rather than the normal rounded shape.	Circulatory disturbance accompanied by angiospasm.
7	Arms	'Drawn in' areas over scapula extending over posterior deltoid.	Circulatory arm and hand problems. Neuritis paraesthesia etc.
8	Head	Thoracic area between scapulae. Lower third of sacrum just above bladder zone. Just below origin of trapezius.	Insomnia and all types of headache. Headaches related to digestive dysfunction. Headaches due to tension.
9	Venous lymphatic disturbance of the legs.	A tight band from middle third of sacrum, parallel to iliac crest laterally and anteriorly over gluteus medius.	Cramp. Swollen legs in summer etc., varicose veins and paraesthesia.

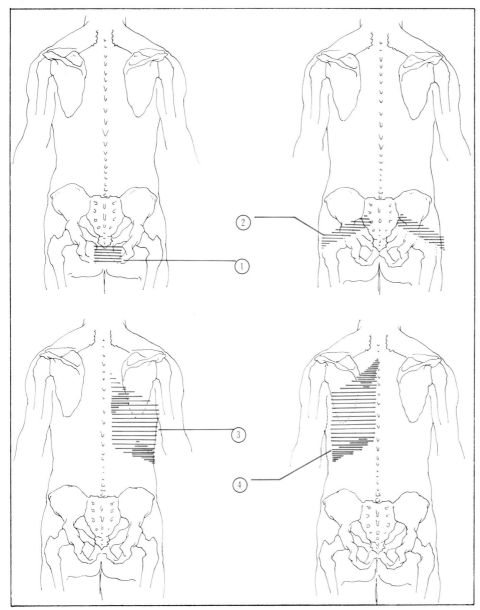

Connective tissue zones (after Ebner). 1. Bladder. 2. Constipation. 3. Liver and Gall
Bladder. 4. Heart.

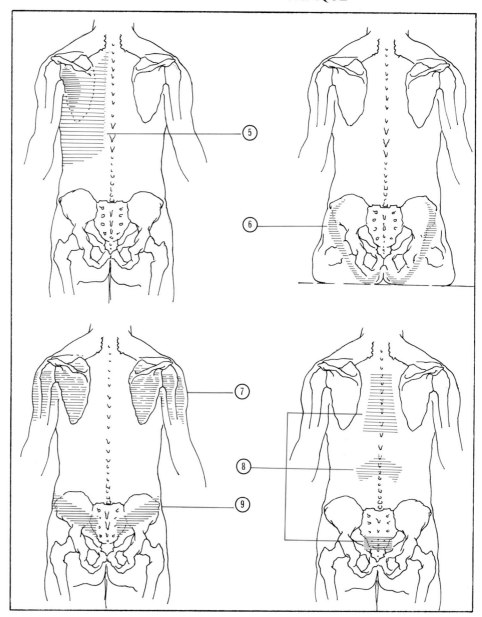

Connective tissue zones (after Ebner). 5. Stomach. 6. Arterial disturbance of the legs. 7. Circulation of arms. 8. Head. 9. Venous lymphatic disturbances of the legs.

With Neuro-muscular Technique these and other areas of soft tissue dysfunction may be found and treated with no obvious symptoms being present. It is clear that tissue changes often precede the appearance of symptoms of underlying pathology and in this alone the diagnostic value of these zones are evident. It is often possible to improve markedly symptoms of organ dysfunction and to improve the function of these organs (liver, stomach etc.) by releasing the congested fibrotic reflex zone. This is not, however, to be considered an end itself since it is clear that underlying causative factors (nutrition, infection etc.) must be dealt with. However, the value of the neuro-muscular tool should not be minimized.

Mackenzie's Abdominal Reflex Areas

Youngs[3] points out that Sir James Mackenzie established a clear relationship between the abdominal wall and the internal abdominal organs. Mackenzie[4] showed that organs which cannot react directly to painful stimuli (i.e. the majority) react by producing spasm and paraesthesia in the reflexly related muscle wall (the moytome) often augmented by hyperaesthesia of the overlying skin (dermatome).

The reflexes involved occur via the autonomic nervous system and can be viscerosomatic *or,* as has been evidenced by many researchers, including Lief, the origin can be somatic and the reflex therefore somatico-visceral.

Mackenzie's abdominal reflex areas are as indicated *(see Figure 3)*. There is sometimes a degree of individualization. However, it is reasonable to state that the presence in abdominal muscles and connective tissues of contracted or sensitive areas indicates (in the absence of recent trauma or strain) some underlying dysfunction which is causing or resulting from the soft tissue lesion.

The reflexes described by Chapman are now commonly termed as neuro-lymphatic reflexes. These can be used in diagnosis and treatment and as a guide to the effectiveness of treatment. In 1965 I described[5] the technique for using these as follows:

Treatment applied through these reflexes, as advocated by Chapman and Owens, consists of a firm but gentle rotary pressure imparted by the index or middle finger. The finger should not be allowed to slip. As these areas are acutely sensitive great care should be taken not to overtreat as the reflex will become fatigued and no benefit will be derived.

My own view coincides with the above method except that I use a variable thumb pressure which fits in with the general neuro-muscular technique. Knowledge of the exact location of the reflexes is of primary importance.

By gentle palpation the operator should first ascertain the presence of involved reflexes. The anterior reflexes should be tested first. If found to be present the anterior reflex should be treated first, then the posterior counterpart of the involved anterior reflexes should be treated. The anterior reflex has, therefore, a dual role, namely, for diagnosis and then to initiate the reflex treatment. The anterior reflex is later of value to ascertain the effectiveness of treatment (after both anterior and posterior reflexes have been treated).

If, on repalpating the reflexes, there is no change in the feel or tenderness, the treatment should be repeated. If there is again no change it indicates either that the pathology is too great for rapid change, or that pathology is irreversible. It may also indicate that some musculoskeletal factor is maintaining the reflex. Primary

Reflex abdominal areas (after Mackenzie). 1. Oesophagus. 2. Stomach. 3. Solar plexus. 4. Spleen. 5. Duodenum. 6. Gall bladder. 7. Ilium. 8. Liver. 9. Caecum and Appendix. 10. Ilium. 11. Ovary and Descending colon. 12. Ureter. 13. Ureter. 14. Colon. 15. Bladder. 16. Ureter.

Figure 3

treatment should then be directed at this factor rather than the reflex. The degree of treatment should be ascertained by palpation. Chapman and Owens described dosage of treatment in terms of seconds, but in practice I feel that anyone experienced in neuro-muscular treatment would have the degree of sensory awareness required to 'feel' when sufficient treatment has been given.

I would stress that I have found the reflexes of Chapman useful in differential diagnosis and in the treatment of various conditions from spastic constipation to migraine—but always as a part of a broad approach to the patient as a whole. That they can influence lymphatic drainage dramatically, I have no doubt—I am less sure of the effect on visceral conditions but have found that the reflexes themselves provide an excellent guide to progress. If they are no longer present then invariably the condition is progressing well.

The illustrations will aid the practitioner in locating these useful diagnostic and therapeutic areas.

Knowledge of Chapman's neuro-lymphatic areas, Mackenzie's reflex areas, connective tissue zones and trigger points might appear a massive task for the memory, and so it is. However, the application of the general knowledge of their existence enables treatment to be effective even without precise knowledge of all the individual reflexes involved. In other words they can be used in diagnosis, if that is the aim. On the other hand they can be treated simply by locating them by palpation and treating whatever is found.

A general neuro-muscular treatment will elicit many such tender areas and the treatment will eliminate a number of them, thus aiding the general body economy. It is not essential, although it is desirable, for the practitioner to know what the various reflex points and areas are. The diagnostic and therapeutic aspects of this method overlap and as a result a number of diagnostic indications will be found in the chapters dealing with treatment. The aim of this chapter has been to try to classify some of the more obvious diagnostic indicators so that the practitioners awareness can be broadened as to the range of diagnostic and therapeutic possibilities.

Etiology

Speransky[6] has stated that the nervous system contains a record of the past history of the organism. The signs present in the musculoskeletal system constitute the map which the practitioner has of past and present dysfunctions. It presents him with the opportunity to treat, alleviate and prevent further dysfunction.

Apart from palpation for tissue changes and reflex trigger areas, diagnosis should involve an evaluation of the gross stress patterns and postural factors. Each patient is an individual challenge and indeed this challenge is renewed at each visit. Thus, whilst the mechanics of treatment are similar the emphasis will probably be different at each visit. It is important that the patient understands this, and the nature of the problem as well as the goal desired. A co-operative patient will accept the time and effort required to achieve that goal.

Observation of the dynamic posture or body in motion gives an idea of balance, posture, gravitational stress, gross structural anomalies etc. Observation of certain body areas in individual movement will then help the visualization of their stress patterns, restrictions etc. Any trained physician, of whatever school, should then be able to decide the direction in which the myofascial tissues require guidance towards the achievement of normal functional integrity. Postural integrity will be considered in a later chapter. The body should also be observed in static positions such as sitting, standing, lying etc.

It is not the role of this work to instruct in postural assessment. The practitioner must learn to appreciate the arrangement of the various body structures and their inter-relationships. The myofascial tensions can then be visualized. When these gross and local postural patterns in active and passive modes have been observed an overall impression can be added to the palpatory impressions, both superficial and deep, which the hands can evaluate with the patient standing, supine or prone. By lightly passing the hands over the various structures alterations in tissue density and configuration can be felt. The deeper palpation to localize the dysfunction can then be performed or left to the neuro-muscular trestment where diagnosis coincides with treatment.

Obviously a history will have been taken prior to observation, palpation, and mobility tests. Such history should be comprehensive and should take note of traumatic incidents, habits, occupational positions and postures, emotional state and history, congenital deformity, surgery and of course general medical history and specific details of the presenting problems.

Mobility tests form, of course, part of the diagnostic procedures in soft tissue assessment. Since all physical therapists are concerned with joint mobility these tests will also be part of any overall assessment. Numerous works exist to instruct in this field.

Active motion, which is movement of one part of the body in relation to another, powered by conscious muscular effort; as well as passive motion in which an outside force acts on the body to induce movement, are both of diagnostic importance. Gradually it is possible to learn to distinguish between healthy tissue and tissue in which there exists dysfunction. This can only be learned by experience.

Observation, static and active; palpation, superficial and deep; a comprehensive and detailed history; mobility tests as required; localization of trigger areas; re-evaluation during the course of treatment; and an intelligent co-operative understanding of the patient and his problems are the diagnostic tools with which to understand the task in hand.

---

[1] Ebner, M., *op. cit.*
[2] Teiriche-Leube, H., *Grundriss der Bindesgewebs Massage* (Fisher, 1960).
[3] Youngs, B., 'NMT of Lower Thorax and Low Back', *British Naturopathic Journal,* Vol. 5, No. 11.
[4] Mackenzie, J., *Symptoms and Their Interpretation* (1909).
[5] Chaitow, Leon, *op. cit.*
[6] Speransky, A. D. *A Basis for the Theory of Medicine* (International Publishers, New York 1943).

Chapter 4

Techniques and Index of
Neurolymphatic Reflexes

The thumb technique employed in NMT enables a wide variety of therapeutic **Thumb**
effects to be produced by its different activities. The tip of the thumb imparts a **Technique**
varying degree of pressure via any of four facets. The very tip may be employed
or the medial or lateral aspect of the tip can be used to make contact with angled
surfaces. For more general (less localized or less specific) contact, of a diagnostic
or therapeutic type, the broad surface of the last phalange of the thumb is often
used.

The hand is always spread so that the direction of the thumb stroke runs
towards one of the fingertips. During the stroke, which covers between two and
three inches (5-8cm), the fingertips act as a fulcrum point. The chief force is
imparted to the thumb tip by the operator leaning onto the thumb in a controlled
manner. The thumb thus never leads the hand but always trails behind the
fingers, the tips of which rest just beyond the end of the stroke.

The extreme versatility of the thumb enables it to modify the direction of
imparted force in accordance with the indications of the tissue being treated. As
the thumb glides across and through those tissues it is an extension of the
operators brain. In fact, for the clearest assessment of what is being palpated the
operator should close his eyes so that every minute change in the tissue can be felt
and reacted to.

The thumb and hand seldom impart their own muscular force except in
dealing with small localized contractures or fibrotic 'nodules'. In order that the
force be transmitted directly to its target, the weight being imparted from the
shoulder should travel in as straight a line as possible. To this end the arm should
not be flexed at the elbow or the wrist by more than a few degrees. The
positioning of the operator's body in relation to the area being treated is also of
the utmost importance in order to facilitate economy of effort and comfort. In
this regard both the optimum height *vis-à-vis* the couch and the most effective
angle of approach to the various body areas must be considered. The
descriptions and illustrations in the treatment sections will aid the operator in
this respect.

The degree of pressure will depend upon the nature of the tissue being treated.
The thumb will allow for a great variety of changes in pressure during its strokes
across and through the tissues. The patient should not feel acute pain but a
general degree of discomfort is usually acceptable as the thumb is seldom

Thumb technique.

Figure 4

stationary. A stroke or glide of two to three inches (5-8cm) will usually take four to five seconds, seldom more unless a particularly obstructive indurated area is being dealt with.

Of course, if reflex pressure techniques are being employed, a much longer stay on a point will be needed, but in normal diagnostic and therapeutic use the thumb continues to move as it probes, decongests and generally treats the tissues. It is not, therefore, possible to state the exact pressures necessary. Obviously on areas with relatively thin muscular covering the pressure would be less than in thick, well covered areas such as the buttocks. Attention should also be paid to the relative sensitivity of different areas and different patients. The thumb is not just mechanically stroked across or through tissue but is an intelligent extension of the operators diagnostic sensitivities and it should feel to the patient as though it is assessing every fibre of his soft tissues. Pain should be transient and no bruising should result if the above advice is followed.

In certain localities the thumb's width prevents the degree of tissue penetration suitable for successful treatment. The middle or index finger can be suitably employed in such areas. The most usual area for this is in the intercostal musculture and in attempting to penetrate beneath the scapula borders in tense fibrotic conditions.

Finger Technique

Figure 5

Finger technique.

The middle finger is slightly flexed and, depending upon the direction of the stroke, is supported by one of its adjacent members. As the treating finger strokes with a firm contact and usually a minimum of lubricant, a tensile strain is created between its tip and the tissue underlying it. This is stretched and lifted by the passage of the finger which, like the thumb, should continue moving unless or until dense, indurated tissue prevents its easy passage. These strokes can be repeated once or twice as tissue changes dictate.

The angle of pressure to the skin surface is between 40° and 50°. The fingertip should never lead the stroke but should always follow the wrist, the palmar surface of which should lead. It is possible to impart a great degree of pull on underlying tissues and the patient's reactions must be taken into account in deciding on the degree of force to be used. Transient pain or marked discomfort are to be expected but no more than that. All sensitive areas are indicative of some degree of dysfunction, local or reflex, and are thus important. This knowledge should be imparted to the patient so that a co-operative attitude is assumed.

Unlike the thumb treatment, in which force is largely directed away from the operator's body, in finger treatment the motive force is usually towards the operator. The arm position therefore alters and a degree of flexion is necessary to ensure that the pull or drag of the finger through the tissues is smooth and in order to protect the hand muscles from strain. Unlike the thumb, which makes a sweep towards the fintertips, whilst the rest of the hand remains relatively stationary, the whole hand will move as the finger pressure is applied. Certainly some variation in the degree of angle between fingertip and skin is allowable during a stroke and some slight variation in the degree of 'hooking' of the finger is sometimes also necessary. However, the main motive force is applied by pulling the slightly flexed middle finger towards the operator with the possibility of some lateral emphasis if needed. The treating finger should always be supported by one of its neighbours, usually the ring finger.

Skin Rolling Technique   This involves the use of either or both hands. The fingers draw tissue towards the operator whilst the ball(s) of the thumb(s) roll over the gathered mound of tissue. In this way the tissue is effectively lifted, stretched and squeezed. The most useful areas of application occur where the tissues lie tight to the underlying structures, such as directly over the shoulder joint and on the lateral aspect of the thigh. The squeezing pressure imparted by the roll of the thumb can be extremely uncomfortable and care should be exercised during its application. The angle of stretch, pull and roll may be varied and repeated several times to impart maximum stimulus to the reflex effects and to stimulate circulation and drainage. Stanley Lief and Boris Chaitow employed this simple, yet effective manoeuvre as part of their general treatment. The latter described its usefulness as follows:

> One of my favourite techniques to enhance nerve and blood circulation is 'skin rolling'. Between the skin and the muscular and bony structures it covers, is a veritable network of blood and nerve structures and functions which can, and often do, fail to achieve their full, effective circulation for high efficiency and health because the skin is often so adhered to its lower structures that circulation and

function is appreciably reduced. This of course adversely affects the efficiency and health of the patient. There is probably no formula that will enhance this aspect of function more effectively than 'skin rolling'. A specific example of its effective benefit is to skin-roll a major joint such as a shoulder in conditions of articular rheumatism, arthritis, neuritis, frozen shoulder etc.

Skin rolling technique.

Figure 6

There are a number of different pressure techniques used for dealing with trigger points. Where underlying (i.e. bony) tissues allow direct pressure onto such points, so that the trigger is squeezed between thumb and the underlying tissue, the variables will be the duration of such pressure and degree of continuous or variable pressure employed. Where no such suitable underlying tissues exist or where it would be dangerous to exert direct pressure through the muscle to the underlying structures (e.g. sternocleidomastoid) then squeezing or pinching techniques are employed. These will also vary with regard to the duration and nature (e.g. variable pressure) of the force imparted.

Pressure Techniques

Chapman suggests a vibratory treatment, lasting ten to fifteen seconds, on the reflexes that he described (neuro-lymphatic). He used fingertip pressure to impart the required energy, although thumb pressure of varying intensity is just as effective. This can be applied as a gradually intensifying pressure building up over five to eight seconds, easing for two or three seconds and then repeated. Altogether this should not take more than half a minute. These points can be over-treated and the optimum time would seem to be from fifteen to thirty seconds with the pressure (or squeeze) of a variable nature. If the patient is able to report a referred pain resulting from the pressure then this can be continued for up to a minute, with fluctuations in the degree of pressure, until the patient indicates a diminution in the referred pain or until the time has elapsed.

It is important to realize that the objective 'feel' of these contractions is unlikely to change during such treatment. Any changes resulting from the treatment will occur later, when homeostatic forces have come into operation. The variation in pressure during the treatment is more desirable than a constantly held degree of pressure, which may irritate and exacerbate the condition. Mitchell, in the Foreword of *An Endocrine Interpretation of Chapman's Reflexes* (Academy of Applied Osteopathy, 1963) recommends that pressure be applied by the pad of the middle finger. This should be maintained as a light direct pressure in an effort to decongest the fluid content of the palpable reflex trigger. Mitchell believes that the determining factor for the amount of treatment to be whether a decrease in oedema takes place or there occurs a dissolution of the gangliform contraction, together with reduction in the sensitivity of the point over a period of between 20 and 120 seconds. The stimuli threshold is being raised in these points and inhibition of noxious impulses is being achieved. There is nothing to be gained from achieving local pressure anaesthesia (numbing) by exaggerated effort. Reflexes that are not painful should not be treated—only an active (and therefore sensitive) reflex point requires attention.

Following treatment of reflex points (trigger points, myofascial triggers, myodysneuria, Chapman's reflexes, etc.) the muscles involved should be actively or passively stretched for up to half a minute each.

Elbow Technique

In treating certain muscle groups, notably the gluteals and the sacrospinalis group, it is sometimes difficult, or impossible, to impart adequate force via the thumb due to the degree of resistance in the tissues involved. Elbow technique treatment should not be given at the same time as NMT but should be preparatory to it, on a number of occasions, so that NMT can subsequently be effectively applied. In treating sacrospinalis, for example, the entire spine should be well lubricated and the operator should stand on the patient's left side (patient supine, pillow under thorax).

The right elbow tip is placed just superior to the sacral base with the forearm at right angles to the patient's body. By flexing the knees slightly and allowing weight to be transferred via the elbow, the operator can apply controlled pressure to the muscles. The elbow is allowed to glide slowly cephalad. If pain is reported, lessen the pressure. Several glides or strokes along the full length of the spine will greatly relax even marked contractions. Similar techniques can be applied to the gluteal area.

Elbow technique.

Figure 7

In using NMT it is often helpful to apply a local 'tissue release' technique to areas of marked contraction or spasticity. In areas overlying bone the techniques suitable for use in the abdominal region are not applicable. The method recommended is as follows:

General, Superficial and Deep Tissue Release Technique

> The contact on the tissues involved is made by extending the digits of either hand and making firm contact with the area between the first and second metacarpo-phalangeal joints. This contact is rotated clockwise or anti-clockwise in order to increase the tension in the underlying tissues. The other hand is then placed over the contact hand so that the downward pressure and rotation are reinforced. In addition, a further direction of stretch should be introduced by the second hand. The tissues are therefore receiving a direct downward pressure, a rotational stretch and a further degree of stretch, all maintained by the two treating hands.

The overlying hand should be placed in such a way that the radial border of the metacarpal base of the thumb is directly over the contact point of the first hand's contact (i.e. over the second metacarpal joint area). The fingers of the overlying hand should be tightly in contact with the lateral border of the contact hand. The final application of the release technique may be performed in one of two ways. The overlying hand executes a short sharp squeeze by flexing the middle finger against the metacarpals of the contact hand. The resulting pressure in the inter-metacarpal area provides the 'thrust' or release force. The line of force of this squeeze is towards the operator.

The second method of release, which is more suitable for deeper contractions of tissue, is applied via short sharp thrust by the overlying hand against the contact hand with a simultaneous medial rotation of the contact hand. The line of force in this technique is away from the operator.

Percussion Technique or Spondylo-therapy

In order to stimulate organs via the spinal pathways, direct percussion techniques have long been employed by Osteopathic and Chiropractic practitioners. A number of mechanical methods exist as does an effective manual system (Gregory's Spondylotherapy).

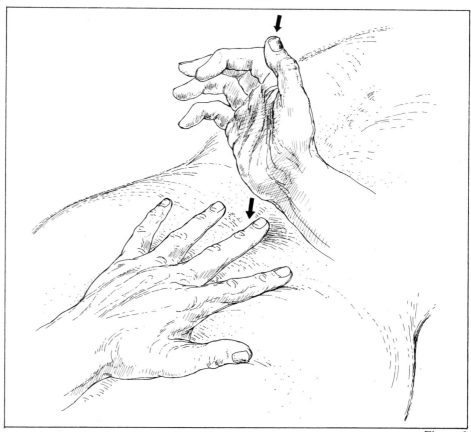

Figure 8

Percussion technique (Spondylotherapy).

The middle finger is placed on the appropriate spinous process and the other hand concusses this with a series of rapidly rebounding blows for approximately five seconds. During this period about fifteen precussive blows should be applied. This technique is usually applied to a series of three or four (or more) adjacent vertebrae. An example of this is the treatment as above, of the fifth thoracic spinous process, proceeding downwards to the ninth, in the case of liver dysfunction. Treatment would only be applied if the area was painful to palpating pressure. Similarly concussion over tenth, eleventh and twelfth thoracic spinous processes would stimulate kidney function.

A mild 'flare up' of symptoms and increased sensitivity in the area treated would normally indicate that the desired degree of stimulation had been achieved. This form of manual spondylotherapy fits into NMT by virtue of its reflex effects and its easy application. Needless to say, a sound knowledge of spinal mechanics and neurological connections is a prerequisite of such a manoeuvre.

Specific Psoas Technique

In postural distortion such as scoliotic or marked lumbar lordotic conditions as well as in many acute low back and sciatic cases, the ilio-psoas muscle is found to be involved.

The Test for Psoas Contraction

Measure for contracted psoas by standing at head of table, with patient lying supine and hands stretched overhead. Be sure to line the mid-line of the palms up with the nose, umbilicus and mid-point between the ankles. Grasp the wrists equally and, with equal tension, pull gently above head as far as possible. The short arm side indicates the side of psoas contraction. Be sure to repeat the test after relaxing psoas. If both arms are found to be of equal length but tension is felt to be equal in both shoulders, then both psoas muscles may be contracted. X-ray diagnosis is the only sure method of determining psoas contraction and its effects on spinal function.

Psoas Technique

(a) Patient lies on back with knees flexed, hands at side. Practitioner stands on side opposite contracted psoas. One hand presses down firmly through the linea alba, three to four inches (7-10cm) below the umbilicus until the probing fingers contact the body of the fourth to fifth lumbars. Then gently slide fingers laterally until the body of the psoas is felt and maintain firm but gentle pressure for about a minute. Check arms overhead and, if even, the psoas is relaxed.

(b) Same as (a) except practitioner is seated on opposite side to contraction. Same contact with fingers through linea alba but with the other hand bringing the flexed leg towards the opposite shoulder and rotating the pelvis against probing fingers.

(c) Same as (a) except the practitioner places his flexed leg on the table to support the patient's leg on contracted psoas side. In this manner, both hands are free to support each other as they penetrate heavier abdomens.

(d) Same as (a) except practitioner's flexed leg supports both patient's legs. This is especially useful when there exists a contraction of both psoas muscles.

Figure 9 (a and b)

Psoas techniques.

Figure 9 (c and d)

Psoas techniques.

Induration Technique

Since many patients are too frail or too ill to allow the full NMT treatment to be applied, a useful technique exists to aid in normalizing reflex and local areas of the para-spinal musculature. Stoddard has pointed out that protective spasm in muscle can often indicate underlying pathology (osteoporosis etc.). Deep pressure techniques would be contra-indicated in such conditions.

With the patient sitting or lying, the operator runs the finger tips longitudinally down the side of the spine over the transverse processes. Any spot or area of hardened or indurated tissue that also palpates as tender to the patient is marked for attention. This is applied by palpating the sensitive area with the tips of the fingers of one hand whilst applying light pressure towards the painful spot with the other hand which is resting on the spinous process of the vertebra alongside the indurated tissue. Direct pressure (light) towards the pain should lessen the degree of tissue contraction and the sensitivity.

If it does not do so then the angle of push on the spinous process towards the painful spot should be varied slightly so that, somewhere within an arc embracing a half circle, an angle of push towards the pain will be found to abolish the pain totally and will lessen the objective feeling of tension. A slightly increased push (not a thrust) is all that is required before moving on to the next indurated area. This technique can be used with NMT or instead of the deeper probing measures which for practical reasons may be contra-indicated (patient's condition or patient's inability to adopt prone position etc.).

Spontaneous Release Technique

In spinal and appendicular strains, injuries or lesions there is often an evident distortion from the normal anatomical posture or position. This eccentric state is often relieved by placing the joint or patient in an exaggerated degree of the deformity found at examination. If this is held for 90 to 120 seconds a spontaneous release will often occur. Jones[1] states that this technique depends on the ability to produce relaxation of reflex muscle tension which limits and binds the joint(s).

The art is in finding the specific direction in which a painful joint can be moved which will release muscular tension and relieve pain. When passively placed in such a position for several minutes a lasting marked inhibition of painful stimuli will result with concomitant increase in motion.

Abdominal Techniques

Boris Chaitow, who worked closely with Lief wrote:

> Stanley Lief taught that manipulation (bony or soft tissue) should not only be confined to the spine itself but also locally to every possible area related to the particular symptom or stress. On the whole the Neuro-muscular Technique he devised is applied with the thumb, as this universally useful digit lends itself to the pattern of pressure and technique required, and is at the same time highly sensitive in diagnostic palpation.
>
> One of the areas of the body which Stanley Lief found uniquely amenable for his soft tissue technique, and can be used with dramatic results, is the abdomen. The enormous variations of functionally and structurally abnormal factors that can develop in the abdominal cavity are manifold. It can be safely asserted that there is no one in middle age and older who has not, unfortunately, developed some of the tensions, contractions, adhesions, nerve and muscle spasms in various parts of the

gastro-intestinal tract and abdominal cavity so common today. All these would normally be outside the scope of the conventional manipulator. But, with the Neuro-muscular Technique, a practitioner can achieve almost dramatic benefits in local stresses and in health in general. He devised for the abdomen the special technique he called 'bloodless surgery' a method of breaking up deep-seated adhesions and contractions. It also enables the operator to improve function and circulation related to female problems such as dysmenorrhoea, menorrhagia and amenorrhoea, fibroids etc.

In developing NMT Stanley Lief displayed an eagerness to learn methods from many sources. He was not content, however, to merely incorporate comple-mentary techniques into his concept but developed and improved on the often crude ideas that others had originated. It was in this refining and adapting process that he showed his genius. During Lief's lifetime, and since his death in 1963, his cousin and former assistant Boris Chaitow has further enlarged on the basic technique and has brought NMT to the point where its application has reached a precise and refined use. As with all manual methods there is an indefinable element of art mixed with the mechanical and scientific aspects of its application. No one can acquire the art without practice and it cannot be taught. The basic mechanics, however, can be passed on by the written word and illustrations or, preferably, by demonstrations.

Specific Abdominal Release Techniques

Lief used methods derived from an American system of manipulative or 'bloodless surgery' to amplify his abdominal techniques. His and Boris Chaitow's technique is presented here. These 'release' techniques can be applied to soft areas of the body (e.g. the throat) as well as to the abdomen. The original concept of 'bloodless surgery' was that adhesions were being 'peeled' away from their anchorage by the technique and in some cases this might have been so. However, its application is to any area of tight, fibrosed, spastic, contracted or adhering soft tissue in the abdominal region. The most dramatic improvements in function are noted after its use in such conditions as spastic or atonic constipation, visceroptosis, dysmenorrhoea, menorrhagia etc. as well as ill-defined abdominal congestion and pain.

Precisely what takes place after release technique is open to conjecture. An improvement in tone and circulation and usually of general function is the most obvious result. It is a matter of debate whether this is because of a release of a long-held contractive state in the soft tissues or because of an actual breaking of adhesions or because of some other mechanism. A general abdominal neuro-muscular treatment precedes the Specific Release Technique A. This serves to both relax and tone the area in a general manner whilst enabling the operator to localize areas which feel indurated or contracted objectively, as well as noting all areas of subjective sensitivity as reported by the patient.

It is these (a) tight, contracted and (b) sensitive areas that receive the release technique. The ability of the operator to localize accurately such areas is obviously critical and must be a matter for constant practice until the hands and fingers feel such abnormalities as a matter of course. To this end it is suggested that the middle finger of the right hand (in a right-handed operator) be trained to seek and mark those areas that will require specific release techniques. This requires practising the use of the hand in a position where the fingers are flexed so that the middle finger is slightly more prominent than its neighbours.

This aids its task of palpating specifically the tissues being probed. The non-searching fingers support the hand and are involved in assessing tissue tension as well as holding movable soft tissues as an aid to the palpating finger. The patient should be supine with knees flexed and feet as close to the buttocks as possible for maximum abdominal relaxation and with the head on a small pillow. The operator should stand facing the patient on the side opposite that being treated, i.e. to treat the left inguinal area the operator stands, knees flexed, leaning across from the patient's right side. This allows the tissues being manipulated to be drawn towards the operator in a controlled manner whereas such a procedure performed with the hands being pushed away from the operator, as would be the case if working from the side being treated, would cause a degree of pushing or gouging of the tissues resulting in pain and a lack of fine control.

Technique A

Having located an area of contracted (often sensitive) tissue the middle finger locates the point of maximum resistance and the tissues are drawn towards the operator, to the limit of pain-free movement. The middle finger and its neighbours should be flexed, fairly rigid and be imparting force in two directions at this stage, i.e. downwards (towards the floor) and towards the operator. (In 'bloodless surgery' techniques the right hand is always on the 'adhesion' and the other contact on the organ to which the lesion is attached.) With the fingers maintaining the above position the thumb of the left hand is placed almost immediately—no more than quarter of an inch (6mm) away—adjacent to the middle finger of the right hand in such a way that a downward pressure (towards the floor) will provide a fulcrum point against which force can be applied via the right hand in order to stretch or reduce the degree of contraction in the tissue (or indeed to break or 'peel' adhesions). The thumb should also be flexed and the contact can be via its tip or its lateral border or a combination of the two.

The idea of a fulcrum is important since the two points of contact are both on soft-tissue structures and the effect of the manipulation is achieved, not by pulling or twisting these apart, but by a combination of movements which impart force in several directions at the same time. This is accomplished by a quick clockwise movement of the right hand (middle finger contact) against the stabilizing anchorage of the left thumb. Movement of the thumb during this release is not essential or necessary. However, Boris Chaitow does impart a degree of additional torsional force by releasing the thumb contact in an anti-clockwise direction at the moment of manipulation.

With both hands in contact, as described, and the contact digits flexed and rigid, the operator should be so positioned that he is leaning over the affected area, knees flexed with the legs separated for stability, elbows flexed and separated to a point of 180° separation. The force that will be present at the point of contact is a downward one, to which is added a slight separation of the hands, which increases the tension on the affected tissues. The manipulative force is imparted by a quick, flicking of the right contact in a clockwise direction whilst maintaining the left thumb contact (or taking it in an anti-clockwise direction).

The effect of the right hand movement would be to snap the right elbow towards the operators side. If a double release is performed then both elbows will

Specific abdominal release techniques.

Figure 10a

come rapidly to the sides. The amount of force imparted should be controlled so that no pain is felt by the patient. The essence of this technique is the speed with which it is applied and its success depends upon this as much as the correct positioning of the hands and the exact location of the area of tissue dysfunction. The same procedure can be repeated several times on the same area and the release of a number of such areas of contracted or indurated tissue, at any one treatment, is usual. The same thumb contact is often maintained whilst variations in the direction of tissue tension are dealt with by slightly altering the angle of the right hand contact and manipulative effort. If, after manipulation, no objective improvement is noted on palpation then the angle of the contacts should be varied. Nothing will be gained, however, by attempting to use excessive force in order to achieve results.

Since the degree of trauma to the patient is minimal, the after-effects should not include bruising of much discomfort. Any such after-effect would indicate undue pressure or force. Boris Chaitow describes the above method as follows:

For the technique of NMT on the abdomen referred to already as 'bloodless surgery' palpate with the tips of the fingers of the right hand, and having located the area of abnormal feel, place those four fingers as a group at the distal border of the lesioned area and place the thumb of the left hand along the nails of the right fingers. Give a sharp flick with both hands simultaneously, the left hand thumb being twisted anticlockwise and the fingers of the right hand clockwise (difficult if not impossible to describe on paper). This achieves an appreciable breaking-up, without trauma or hurt to the patient, of tensions, adhesions, congestions etc., both on the wall of the abdomen and structures within the cavity. Obviously these flicks with the hands have to be repeated a number of times to feel a discernible difference in the lesioned tissue. Stanley Lief achieved dramatic changes in tissue structure and functional improvements in many types of abdominal stresses including digestive problems, gall bladder blockage, gall stones, constipation, spastic colon, colic, colitis, uterine fibroids, dysmenorrhoea, menorrhagia, small non-malignant abdominal tumours, post-operative adhesions etc.

Technique B
A second method for the release of tense, contracted, indurated connective and muscular tissue, is sometimes employed. This requires the same positioning of the patient and the operator, as in method A. It is worth recalling that thickening will occur in fascia in accordance with the degree of stress imposed upon it. Since enormous gravitational stress occurs in the abdominal region, as a result of postural embarrassment, it is frequently the case that tight 'stress bands' will be felt inferior, superior or lateral to internal organs (e.g. intestinal structures) that have sagged and become displaced. Such contracted tissue is often the source of reflex trigger activity and is often, in itself, the cause of mechanical interference with normal venous and lymphatic drainage as well as being a possible source of pain. Any procedure that helps to normalize such tension should be accompanied by a programme of postural re-education and exercise if it is to have any lasting beneficial effects.

The operator's right hand, fingers flexed and middle finger slightly in the lead, probes through the surface abdominal musculature and attempts to 'lift' the structures beneath towards himself. In this way, areas of abnormal resistance will be quite easily traced by the tip of the middle finger of the right hand. The most inferior point of attachment of such a band is located and held firmly by this flexed digit. The tip and lateral border of the thumb of the left hand is then placed adjacent to this contact so that the right hand contact is on the tension band and the left contact is on the structure to which it attaches. The manipulative force is achieved by a rapid, anticlockwise movement of the right contact whilst firm, stabilizing pressure is maintained by the left thumb.

The closer the two contacts are to each other at the moment of release, the less force is required and the less danger of injury to the tissues there will be. It is suggested that by visualizing an attempt to tear an envelope held between thumbs and forefingers this concept will be better understood. The closer the holding digits are to each other the easier such an operation would be. Since the manipulative effort is attempting to, at least, stretch and, at most, separate the fibres involved it is necessary to impart a high velocity, low amplitude torsional force and not a vague stretching effort imparted over a large area of unyielding tissue.

The actual manipulative force is imparted by the tip of the middle finger of the right hand but is of course the result of the movement of the whole hand. The

Specific abdominal release techniques.   *Figure 10b*

wrist snaps medially and the elbow outwards at the moment of release. This speedy 'flicking' action is one that should be practised over and over again so that its execution is a matter of routine. A release of contracted tissue will be followed by an immediate freedom of mobility of tissues and of organs formerly 'bound' and immobile. Such 'release' procedures (A or B) should be performed throughout the abdominal area and should be preceded by the general neuro-muscular treatment and be followed by a general procedure to 'lift' the abdominal contents back to a physiologically correct position. Abdominal and postural exercises on the part of the patient, combined with diaphragmatic breathing techniques, should also be carried out. A series of six to ten such treatments over a period of a month or so is suggested in chronic conditions involving visceroptosis and abdominal congestion. The application of these techniques to the hypogastric and inguinal regions will be found to be of immense benefit to patients suffering from menstural irregularities. Local function will be greatly improved as a result of the structural and circulatory improvements following specific release techniques.

'S' Contact Technique   The hands should be positioned in such a way as to allow basic thumb technique to be applied across the fibres of a contracted or indurated muscle or soft tissue area so that the thumbs are travelling in opposite directions to each other, about one inch apart. In this way, as the short stroke is applied simultaneously with each thumb at a slow speed, the tissues between the two thumbs will be progressively stretched. This technique should be applied along the course of particularly spastic and hard unyielding tissues, as well as the basic thumb technique. It is called 'S' contact because the tissues being treated form that shape as the strokes are performed. The same procedure exactly may be used, but with a flicking action of the thumb to complete the stroke, once effective tension has been created in the tissues by the opposing thumbs. This 'springing' has the effect of stimulating local circulation most effectively and if the tissues are not too sensitive, may be effective in breaking down infiltrated or indurated tissues.

Piriformis Muscle Technique   The piriformis muscle syndrome results from contracture of the muscle which is usually traumatic in origin. The effects can be circulatory, neurological and functional, inducing pain and paraesthesia of the affected limb as well as alterations to pelvic and lumbar function. Diagnosis usually hinges on the absence of spinal causative factors and the distributions of symptoms from the sacrum to the hip joint, over the gluteal region and down to the popliteal space. Palpation of the affected piriformis tendon, near the head of the trochanter will elicit pain. The affected leg will be externally rotated.

The piriformis muscle syndrome is frequently characterized by such bizarre symptoms that they may seem unrelated. One characteristic complaint is a persistent, severe, radiating low-back pain extending from the sacrum to the hip joint, over the gluteal region and the posterior portion of the upper leg, to the popliteal space. In the most severe cases the patient will be unable to lie or stand comfortably, and changes in position will not relieve the pain. Intense pain will occur when the patient sits or squats since this type of movement requires external rotation of the upper leg and flexion at the knee.

A common sign of the piriformis syndrome is a persistent external rotation of the upper leg. This indication, which is known as the positive piriformis sign, is easily detected when the patient is examined in the supine position.

The buttock on the same side as the piriformis lesion is usually sensitive to touch or palpation. Severe pain may occur when pressure is applied to the area over the piriformis muscle and its tendinous insertion on the head of the greater trochanter.

Another diagnostic sign may be the shortening of the leg on the affected side due to contracture of the piriformis muscle. In cases where the leg on the opposite side appears shortened, it is probable that some other dysfunction exists and that the condition is not directly related to the piriformis syndrome.

In order to determine the effects of a piriformis muscle contracture on the sacrum, the patient should be examined in the prone position. In the case of a right piriformis muscle contracture, there will be a left oblique axis rotation of the sacrum. The sacral base on the right side will be seen to be anterior in relation to the posterior, superior iliac spine. The sulcus overlying this spine will be deepened because of the anterior rotation of the sacrum. The apex of the sacrum will be found to have moved to the left of the midline and more posteriorly at the level of the posterior inferior spine of the ilium. The sulcus on the left side will appear to be shallow because of the posterior movement of the sacrum at this point.

Additional findings that result from this oblique axis rotation of the sacrum include rotoscoliosis of the lumbar vertebrae and increased lordosis. There may be secondary or multiple lesion patterns that affect the entire vertebral column, including the atlanto-occipital region.

The patient also may mention pain that follows the distribution pattern of the sciatic nerve to the level of the popliteal space and sometimes to the more distal branches of this nerve. When the common perineal nerve is involved, there may be a paraesthesia of the posterior surface of the upper leg and some portions of the lower leg.

One of the most perplexing problems arising from the piriformis syndrome is the involvement of the pudendal nerve and blood vessels. This nerve with its branches, provides the major sensory innervation of the perineal skin and the somatic motor innervation of much of the external genitalia and related perineal musculature in both women and men. The pudendal blood vessels supply essentially the same areas. The pudendal nerve, after passing through the greater sciatic foramen, re-enters the pelvis by way of the lesser sciatic foramen. As it proceeds, it divides into three main branches. These are the inferior heamorrhoidal nerve, the perineal nerve, and the dorsal nerve to the clitoris (or penis). The perineal nerve divides into the posterior labia majora (or the scrotum) and the perineal body. The deep branch of the perineal nerve supplies the levator ani (in part), the transversus perinei superficialis and profundus, the bulbocavernosus, and the ischiocavernosus muscles. The branch to the bulbocavernosus further divides to supply the bulb. The dorsal nerve to the clitoris also supplies the crura, the prepuce, and the glans of the clitoris (or penis).

Compression of the pudendal nerve and blood vessels can result in serious problems involving the functioning of the genitalia in both sexes. Since external rotation of the upper legs is required for women during coitus, if there were interference with the blood supply and innervation of the genitalia, it is understandable that a female patient might complain of pain during sexual intercourse. This could also be a basis for impotency in men.

Thumb pressure is sufficient to remedy the problem which might require manipulation but which often yields to the following treatment.

Patient lying on side, affected side uppermost, legs flexed at hip and knees. The operator's elbow is applied to the piriformis tendon and heavy downward pressure is exerted for ten seconds at a time, up to ten times, with a few seconds rest in between. This should relieve symptoms of a traumatic nature where the condition is not of too long standing and where no spinal or sacro-iliac involvement is present. *(See Figure 11a.)*

With Te Poorten's approach to piriformis contracture the patient lies on the non-affected side with the knees flexed and the upper legs perpendicular to the body. The operator places his elbow on the piriformis musculo-tendinous junction and a steady pressure of 20-30 lbs (9-13kg) is applied. With his other hand he abducts the foot so that it will force an internal rotation of the upper leg.

Figure 11 (a and b)

Piriformis techniques.

Figure 11 (c and d)

Piriformis techniques.

The leg is held in the rotated position for periods of up to two minutes. This procedure is repeated to or three times. The patient is then placed in the supine position and the affected leg is tested for freedom of both external and internal rotation. *(See Figures 11b and 11c)*

The second stage of treatment is performed with the patient in the supine position with both legs extended. The foot of the affected leg is grasped and the leg is flexed at both the knee and the hip. At the same time the foot is turned inward, which forces an external rotation of the upper leg. When the operator causes the patient's leg to be extended, the foot is turned outward, resulting in an internal rotation of the upper leg. During the procedure the patient is instructed to resist the movements; this accomplishes a modified form of isometric activity of the muscles. This treatment method, repeated two or three times, also serves to relieve the contracture of the muscles of external and internal rotation. *(See Figure 11d)*

Vapo-coolant Technique

The following method is adapted from the work of Dr's Travell and Mennell[?] In the first place, one should use a container of vapo-coolant spray with a calibrated nozzle which delivers a moderately fine jet stream. The jet stream should have sufficient force to carry in the air for at least three feet. A mist-like spray is less desirable.

The patient should be comfortably supported to promote muscular relaxation. The container is held about two feet away, in such a manner that the jet stream meets the body surface at an acute angle or at a tangent, not perpendicularly. This lessens the shock of the impact. For the same reason, the stream is sometimes started in air or on the operator's hand and is gradually brought into contact with the skin overlying the trigger point.

The stream is applied in one direction, not back and forth. Each sweep is started at the trigger point and is moved slowly and evenly outward over the reference zone. Probably it is advantageous to spray both trigger and reference areas, since secondary trigger points are likely to have developed within reference zones when pain is very strong. (The direction of movement is also in line with the muscle fibres towards their insertion.)

The optimum speed of movement of the sweep over the skin seems to be about four inches (10cm) per second. Sweeps are repeated in a rhythm of a few seconds on and a few seconds off, until all of the skin over trigger and reference areas has been covered once or twice. If aching or 'cold pain' develops, or if the application of the spray sets off a reference of pain, the interval between sweeps is lengthened. Care is taken not to frost or blanch the skin.

During the sweeps, appropriate passive assisted motion should be employed to stretch gently the muscle containing the trigger point. Steady, gentle stretching is usually essential if a satisfactory result is to be achieved. As relaxation occurs, continued stretch should be maintained.

After each series of sweeps, active motion is tested. The patient is asked to move in the directions which were restricted before spraying was begun. An attempt should be made to restore the full range of motion, but always within the limits of pain, since sudden over-stretching increases existing muscle spasm. At the same time precautions are taken not to strain the muscles under treatment, either then or during the next few days.

The treatment is continued in this manner until the trigger points (several are usually present) and their respective pain reference zones have been sprayed. The entire procedure may occupy fifteen or twenty minutes, and cannot be carried out properly if rushed. However, after spraying the first trigger point for a minute or two and testing it for changes in sensitivity to pressure, one can usually predict whether a successful result will be obtained with the technique. Simple exercises which utilize the principle of passive stretch should be outlined to the patient, to be carried out several times daily, after the application of gentle heat (hot packs etc.).

The importance of re-establishing normal motion in conjunction with the use of the vapo-coolant spray is well founded. It may be that the brief interruption by the spray of the stream of pain impulses is not enough and that the input of normal impulses must also be achieved for the successful obliteration of the trigger points to be achieved.

All the methods described in this chapter may be incorporated into general Neuro-muscular Technique treatment.

Technique for Neuro-lymphatic Reflexes (Chapman's Reflexes) and Index to Illustrations

The reflexes may be treated as part of a general neuro-muscular treatment or on their own in accordance with the recommendations contained in Mitchell's *An Endocrine Interpretation of Chapman's Reflexes*. This advises the treating by light digital pressure of the anterior reflex followed by the corresponding posterior reflex. The anterior point should then be re-examined and if there has been a palpable change, or if sensitivity has diminished, then no more action would be required. If no such change is found then the treatment to the anterior and then the posterior points is again carried out and if still no change is noted then it is assumed that pathology is too great for a rapid change or is irreversible or that there is a musculoskeletal factor maintaining the dysfunction. If this approach is adopted then the grouping of reflexes into systems is a useful method. If one of a group is found to be active then all others in the group should be examined and, if active, treated; for example, the endocrine group comprises: prostate, gonads, broad ligaments, uterus, thyroid and adrenals.

The gastro-intestinal group comprises the colon, thyroid, pancreas, duodenum, small intestine and liver. The infections group comprises liver, spleen and the adrenals. The advice therefore is to use reflexes intelligently, treating only what is palpable and sensitive.

Some of the anterior reflexes (the ones which should, in theory, be treated first, lie on the posterior aspect of the body. These include those for haemorrhoids (No. 48) and cerebellar congestion (No. 21) and leucorrhoea (No. 25) and salpingitis (No. 41).

It is suggested that reference be made to the above-mentioned book for more detailed study. The notes following give the reflex by name, number and description of location together with an indication of which drawing illustrates it. It was not found to be possible to incorporate all the drawings onto one picture without creating a confusing series of overlaps. It is suggested that the practitioner learns to search appropriate areas for the type of sensitive tissue changes which are the manifestation of these reflexes and to use the drawings and the following list to become familiar with the patterns and groups of these important aids to healing.

[1] Jones, L. H., 'Foot Treatment Without Hand Trauma', *Journal of the American Osteopathic Association* (January, 1963).
[2] Mennell, J., 'Therapeutic Use of Cold', *Journal of the American Osteopathic Association,* Vol. 74, No. 12.
Travell, Dr J., 'Ethyl Chloride Spray for Painful Muscle Spasm', *Arch. Phys. Med. Rehabl.* 33 pp. 291-8 (May, 1952).

Table 3. Location of Reflexes

Reflex No.	Symptoms or Area	Anterior	Figure	Posterior	Figure
1	Conjunctivitis and retinitis	Upper humerus	12a	Occipital area	12c
2	Nasal problems	Anterior aspect of first rib close to sternum.	12a	Posterior to angle of the jaw on the tip of the transverse process of the first cervical vertebra.	12c
3	Arms (circulation)	Muscular attachments of pectoralis minor to third, fourth and fifth ribs.	12a	Superior angle of scapula and superior third of the medial margin of the scapula.	12c
4	Tonsilitis	Between first and second ribs close to sternum.	12a	Midway between spinous process and tip of transverse process of first cervical vertebra.	12d
5	Thyroid	Second intercostal space close to sternum.	12a	Midway between spinous process and tip of transverse process of second thoracic vertebra.	12c
6	Bronchitis	Second intercostal space close to sternum.	12a	Midway between spinous process and tip of transverse process of second thoracic vertebra.	12d
7	Oesophagus	As No. 6.	12a	As No. 6	12d
8	Myocarditis	As No. 6.	12a	Between the second and third thoracic transverse processes. Midway between the spinous process and the tip of the transverse process.	12d
9	Upper Lung	Third intercostal space close to the sternum.	12a	As No. 8.	12d
10	Neutritis of upper limb	As No. 9.	12a	Between the third and fourth transverse processes, midway between the spinous process and the tip of the transverse process.	12d
11	Lower Lung	Fourth intercostal space, close to sternum.	12a	Between fourth and fifth transverse processes. Midway between the spinous process and the tip of the transverse process.	12d

Reflex No.	Symptoms or Area	Anterior	Figure	Posterior	Figure
12	Small intestines	Eighth, ninth and tenth intercostal spaces close to cartilage.	12a	Eighth, ninth and tenth thoracic intertransverse spaces.	12c
13	Gastric hyper-congestion	Sixth intercostal space to the left of the sternum.	12a	Sixth thoracic-intertransverse space, left side.	12c
14	Gastric hyperacidity	Fifth intercostal space to the left of the sternum	12a	Fifth thoracic intertranverse space, left side.	12e
15	Cystitis	Around the umbilicus and on the pubic symphysis close to the midline.	12a	Upper edge of the transverse processes of the second lumbar vertebra.	12e
16	Kidneys	Slightly superior to and lateral to the umbilicus.	12a	In the interverse space between the twelfth thoracic and the first lumbar vertebra.	12e
17	Atonic constipation	Between the anterior superior spine of the ilium and the trochanter.	12a	Eleventh costal vertebral junction.	12c
18	Abdominal tension	Superior border of the pubic bone.	12a	Tip of the transverse process of the second lumbar vertebra.	12d
19	Urethra	Inner edge of pubic ramus near superior aspect of symphysis.	12a	Superior aspect of transverse process of second lumbar vertebra.	12e
20	Depuytrens contracture, and arm and shoulder pain	None	—	Anterior aspect of lateral margin of scapulae, inferior to the head of humerus.	12e
21	Cerebral congestion (related to paralysis or paresis).	(On the posterior aspect of the body.) Lateral from the spines of the third, fourth and fifth cervical vertebrae.	12a	Between the transverse processes of the first and second cervical vertebrae.	12d
22	Clitoral irritation and vaginismus	Upper medial aspect of the thigh.	12a	Lateral to the junction of the sacrum and the coccyx.	12d
23	Prostate	Lateral aspect of the thigh from the trochanter to just above the knee. Also lateral to symphysis pubis as in uterine conditions (see No. 43).	12a	Between the posterior superior spine of the ilium and the spinous process of the fifth lumbar vertebra.	12d

Reflex No.	Symptoms or Area	Anterior	Figure	Posterior	Figure
24	Spastic constipation or colitis	Within an area of an inch or two wide extending from the trochanter to within an inch of the patella.	12a	From the transverse processes of the second, third and fourth lumbar vertebrae to the crest of the ilium.	12c
25	Leucorrhoea	Lower medial aspect of thigh, slightly posteriorly (on the posterior aspect of the body).	12a & 12c	Between the posterior superior spine of the ilium and the spinous process of the fifth lumbar vertebra.	12d
26	Sciatic neuritis	Anterior and posterior to the tibiofibula junction.	12a	1. On the sacroiliac synchondrosis. 2. Between the ischial tuberosity and the acetabulum. 3. Lateral and posterior aspects of the thigh.	12c
27	Torpid liver (nausea, fullness malaise)	Fifth intercostal space, from the mid-mammillary line to the sternum.	12b	Fifth thoracic intertransverse space on the right side.	12c
28	Cerebellar congestion (memory and concentration laspses).	Tip of coracoid process of scapula.	12b	Just inferior to the base of the skull on the first cervical vertebra.	12d
29	Otitis media	Upper edge of clavicle where it crosses the first first rib.	12b	Superior aspect of first cervical transverse process (tip).	12c
30	Pharyngitis	Anterior aspect of the first rib close to the sternum.	12b	Midway between the spinous process and the tip of the transverse process of the second cervical vertebra.	12d
31	Laryngitis	Upper surface of the second rib, two or three inches (5-8cm) from the sternum.	12b	Midway between the spinous process and the tip of the second cervical vertebra.	12d
32	Sinusitis	Lateral to the sternum on the superior edge of the second rib in the first intercostal space.	12b	As No. 31.	12d
33	**Pyloric stenosis**	On the sternum.	12b	Tenth costovertebral junction on the right side.	12e

Reflex No.	Symptoms or Area	Anterior	Figure	Posterior	Figure
34	Neurasthenia	All the muscular attachments of pectoralis major on the humerus clavicle, sternum, ribs (especially fourth rib).	12b	Below the superior medial edge of the scapula on the the face of the fourth rib.	12d
35	Wry Neck (Torticollis)	Medial aspect of the upper edge of the humerus.	12b	Transverse processes of the third, fourth, sixth and seventh cervical vertebrae.	12d
36	Splenitis	Seventh intercostal space close to the cartilagenous junction, on the left.	12b	Seventh intertransverse space on the left.	12c
37	Adrenals (allergies, exhaustion, etc.)	Superior and lateral to umbilicus.	12b	In the intertransverse space between the eleventh and twelfth thoracic vertebrae.	·12e
38	Mesoappendix	Superior aspect of the twelfth rib, close to the tip, on right.	12b	Lateral aspect of the eleventh intercostal space on the right.	12c
39	Pancreas	Seventh intercostal space on the right, close to the cartilage.	12b	Seventh thoracic intertransverse space on the right.	12e
40	Liver and gall bladder congestion	Sixth intercostal space, from the mid-mammillary line to the sternum (right side).	12a & 12b	Sixth thoracic intertransverse space, right side.	12e
41	Salpingitis or vesiculitis	Midway between the acetabulum and the sciatic notch (this is on the posterior aspect of the body).	12e	Between the posterior, superior spine of the ilium and the spinous process of the fifth lumbar vertebra.	12d
42	Ovaries	The round ligaments from the superior border of the pubic bone, inferiorly.	12b	between the ninth and tenth intertransverse space and the tenth and eleventh intertransverse space.	12d
43	Uterus	Anterior aspect of the junction of the ramus of the pubis and the ischium.	12b	Between the posterior superior spine of the ilium and the fifth lumbar spinous process.	12d
44	Uterine fibroma	Lateral to the symphysis, extending diagonally inferiorly.	12b	Between the tip of the transverse process of the fifth lumbar vertebra and the crest of the ilium.	12c

flex o.	Symptoms or Area	Anterior	Figure	Posterior	Figure
5	Rectum	Just inferior to the lesser trochanter.	12b	On the sacrum close to the ilium at the lower end of the iliosacral synchondrosis.	12e
6	Broad ligament (uterine involvement usual).	Lateral aspect of the thigh from the trochanter to just above the knee.	12b	Between the posterior, superior spine of the ilium and the fifth lumbar spinous process.	12d
7	Groin glands (circulation and drainage of legs and pelvic organs).	Lower quarter of the sartorius muscle and its attachment to the tibia.	12b	On the sacrum close to the ilium at the lower end of iliosacral synchondrosis.	12e
8	Haemorrhoids	Just superior to the ischial tuberosity. (These areas are on the posterior surface of the body.)	12d	On the sacrum close to the ilium, at the lower end of the iliosacral synchondrosis.	12d
9	Tongue	Anterior aspect of second rib at the cartilaginous junction with the sternum.	12a	Midway between the spinous process and the tip of the transverse process of the second cervical vertebra.	12d

Chapman's neuro-lymphatic reflexes.

Chapman's neuro-lymphatic reflexes.

Chapman's neuro-lymphatic reflexes.

Figure 12d

Chapman's neuro-lymphatic reflexes.

Figure 12e

Chapman's neuro-lymphatic reflexes.

Chapter 5

Basic Spinal
Neuro-muscular Technique

The objectives to which the practitioner's efforts are aimed may include postural reintegration, tension release, pain relief, improvement of joint mobility, reflex stimulation or sedation. There exist a great number of variations to the basic technique as developed by Stanley Lief. Some of these variations will depend upon the particular presenting factors and others upon personal preference on the part of the practitioner. As with all areas of therapy, ideas and techniques have been borrowed from other systems and incorporated into the overall technique. This is valid if these methods fit into the philosophical and practical framework of NMT. Similarities between some aspects of NMT and other manual systems should therefore be anticipated.

What is unique to NMT is its concentration on the soft tissues, not just to give reflex benefit to the body, not just to prepare for other therapeutic methods such as exercise or manipulation, not just to relax and normalize tense fibrotic muscular tissue and not just to enhance lymphatic and general circulation and drainage, but to do all these things and, at the same time, to give the practitioner diagnostic information via the palpating and treating instrument which is usually the hand and, more specifically, the thumb.

The technique can be applied generally or locally and in a variety of positions (sitting, lying etc.). The order in which body areas are dealt with is not regarded as critical in general treatment but is of some consequence in postural reintegration.

The basic spinal NMT treatment and the basic abdominal (and related areas) NMT treatment are the most commonly used and will be our first consideration. The methods described are in essence those of Stanley Lief and Boris Chaitow, both of whom achieved (and in the latter case continue to achieve) a degree of skill in the application of NMT that is unsurpassed. The inclusion of data on reflex areas and effects, together with basic NMT methods, provides the operator with a useful therapeutic tool, the limitations of which will be largely determined by the degree of intelligence and understanding with which it is employed. As Boris Chaitow has written:

The important thing to remember is that this unique manipulative formula is applicable to *any* part of the body for *any* physical and physiological dysfunction and for both articular and soft tissue lesions.

The learner should begin to develop the art of palpation and sensitivity of fingers by constantly feeling the appropriate areas and assessing any abnormality in tissue structure for tensions, contractions, adhesions, spasms etc.

It is important to acquire with practice an appreciation of the 'feel' of *normal* tissue so that one is better able to recognize abnormal tissue. Once some level of diagnostic sensitivity with fingers has been achieved, subsequent application of the technique will be much easier to develop. The whole secret is to be able to recognize the 'abnormalities' in the feel of tissue structures. Having become accustomed to understanding the texture and character of 'normal' tissue, the pressure applied by the thumb in general, especially in the spinal structures, should always be firm, but never hurtful or bruising. To this end the pressure should be applied with a 'variable' pressure, i.e. with an appreciation of the texture and character of the tissue structures and according to the feel that sensitive fingers should have developed. The level of the pressure applied should not be consistent because the character and texture of tissue is always variable. These variations can be detected by one's educated 'feel'. The pressure should, therefore, be so applied that the thumb is moved along its path of direction in a way which corresponds to the feel of the tissues.

This variable factor in finger pressure constitutes probably the most important quality an operator of NMT can learn, enabling him to maintain more effective control of pressure, develop a greater sense of diagnostic feel, and be far less likely to bruise the tissue.

Use of Lubricant

The use of a lubricant to facilitate the smooth passage of, for example, the thumb over the surface is an essential aspect of NMT. However, at times the degree of stimulus imparted via the tissues can be enhanced by increasing the tensile strain between the thumb or finger and the skin.

If this effect is required, notably to achieve a rapid vascular response, then no lubricant should be used. Similar reactions will be achieved (with lubricant) where NMT is applied along the intermuscular septa or at the origins and insertions of muscles.

The lubricant used should not allow too slippery a passage of the operating digit. A mixture of two parts rape seed oil to one part lime water provides a suitable degree of lubrication. It should be clear to the operator that underlying tissues being treated should be visualized and, depending upon the presenting symptoms and the area involved, any of a number of procedures may be undertaken as the hand moves from one site to another. There may be superficial stroking in the direction of lymphatic flow, or direct pressure along the line of axis of stress fibres, or deeper alternating 'make and break' stretching and pressure or traction on fascial tissue. At the same time, diagnostic information is being received and this determines the variations in pressure and the direction of force being applied. Such changes must take place without the sudden release or application of force which could irritate the patient and produce violent pains and contraction.

Lief's basic spinal treatment followed the pattern as set out below. The fact that the same pattern is followed at each treatment does not mean that the treatment is necessarily the same. The pattern gives a framework and a useful starting and ending point, but the degree of emphasis applied to the various areas of dysfunction that manifest themselves is a variable factor which makes each treatment different. The areas of dysfunction should be recorded on a case card together with all relevant material and diagnostic findings. The myofascial tissue changes, trigger points and reference zones, areas of sensitivity, restricted motion etc. should all be recorded and referred to at each visit.

Appropriate notes should be made after each visit as to changes in these factors as well as details of the treatment given. To this end a system of 'shorthand' is desirable so that the practitioner can speedily note and decipher the essential elements of a particular visit. A code can be developed to record the patient's observations about the progress made after the previous treatment, e.g. OOX might be used to indicate improvement for the first two weeks after treatment followed by a return of symptoms and XOX might be used to indicate an initial worsening, followed by an improvement and then a deterioration.

To this end the following symbols might be applied: X indicates deterioration; = indicates the same; O indicates improvement. In noting the actual treatment applied the following examples might be instructive. Sp. NMT esp. C1,2 (R). D2,3 (R) + ICS 2,3 and 4(R). LDJ. TFL X2, indicates spinal neuro-muscular technique especially first and second cervical on the right, second and third dorsal on the right, second, third and fourth intercostal spaces on the right, lumbo dorsal junction, tensor fascia lata (both). This would indicate the areas of main fibrotic change or sensitivity. Also to be noted are trigger areas and reflex zones. For example, P° and str. to L/st-mast ★ pt. indicates pressure and stretch technique left sterno-mastoid trigger point.

These examples are meant to encourage the practitioner to keep accurate records. Ideally a universal shorthand would enhance the interchange of information between practitioners. However, what really matters is that the individual understands and refers to his own well-kept records. In this way useful information and patterns of clinical interest can become apparent to the research-minded practitioner. Invariably when, due to pressure of work, there is a lapse of concentration and the notes of a particular treatment are scanty or even missing, the patient will report an interesting development or improvement and the practitioner is left wondering what it was that achieved the change. The development of a personal shorthand to cover all treatment given, whether manipulative, soft tissue, exercise, or any other modality, is an essential aspect of successful case management.

Lief's Basic Spinal Treatment

Lief's basic spinal NMT treatment follows a pattern of placing the patient prone with a medium pillow under the chest, forehead supported by the patient's hands or ideally resting in a split headpiece. The whole spine from occiput to sacrum, including the gluteal area is lightly oiled. The operator should begin by standing half-facing the head of the couch on the left of the patient with his hips level with the mid thoracic area. In order to facilitate the intermittent application of pressure and the transfer of weight via the arm to the exploring and treating thumb, the practitioner should stand with the left foot forward of the right by 12-18 inches (30-45cm), his weight evenly distributed between them, knees slightly flexed.

The first contact is a gliding, light-pressured movement of the medial tip of the right thumb, from the mastoid process along the nuchal line to the external occipital protuberance. This same stroke, or glide, is then repeated with deeper pressure. The movement of the thumb through the tissue is slow, not uniformly slow, but deliberately seeking and feeling for contractions and congestions (to use two words which will be meaningful to any manual therapist). If and when such localized areas are felt the degree of pressure is increased and, in a variably applied manner, this pressure carries the thumb tip across or through the restricting tissue.

It is almost impossible to describe in words what this should feel like to the practitioner let alone the patient. The patient will often report a degree of pain but may say that it 'feels good'. It is a contradiction in terms, but constructive pain is usually felt as a 'nice hurt'.

Practitioner's Posture   The treating arm should not be flexed, since the optimum transmission of weight from the operator's shoulder, through the arm to the thumb tip, is best achieved with a relatively straight arm. This demands that the practitioner ensures that the plinth height is suitable for his own height. Thus, he should not be forced to stand on tip-toe to treat his patient, nor should he have to adopt an unhealthy bent posture. The operator's weight should be evenly spread between his separated feet, both of which are forward facing at this stage. In this way, by slightly altering his own weight distribution from the front to the back foot, and vice-versa, an accurate, controlled degree of pressure can be exerted with minimum arm or hand effort.

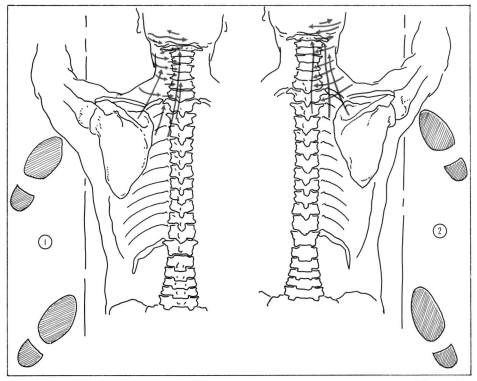

Figure 13a

Neuro-muscular Technique. Illustrating position of operator and lines of application.

The hand itself should not be rigid but in a relaxed state, moulding itself to the contours of the neck or back tissues. To some extent the fingertips stabilize the hand. The thumb's glide is controlled by this so that the actual stroke is achieved by the tip of the extended thumb being brought slowly across the palm towards the fingertips. The fingers during this phase of cervical treatment would be placed on the opposite side of the neck to that being treated. The fingers maintain their position as the thumb performs its therapeutic glide. The illustrations will aid the reader to a better understanding of this description.

Were all the effort to be on the part of the thumb it would soon tire. What has to be learned is that whilst the transverse movement of the thumb is a hand or forearm effort and the relative straightness or rigidity of the last two thumb segments is also a local muscular responsibility, the vast majority of the energy imparted via the thumb results from the practitioner's body position. Increase in pressure can be speedily achieved by simple weight transfer from back towards front foot and a slight 'lean' onto the thumb from the shoulders.

The first two strokes of the right thumb having been completed—one shallow and almost totally diagnostic and the second, deeper, imparting therapeutic effort, the next stroke is half a thumb width caudal to the first. Thus a degree of overlap occurs as these strokes, starting on the belly of the sterno-cleidomastoid, glide across and through the trapezius, splenius capitus and posterior cervical muscles. A progressive series of strokes is applied in this way until the level of the cervico-dorsal junction is reached. Unless serious underlying dysfunction is found it is seldom necessary to repeat the two superimposed strokes at each level of the cervical region.

If underlying fibrotic tissue appears unyielding a third or fourth slow, deep, glide may be necessary. The degree of discomfort engendered in the patient is of some importance. The sensitivity of this region is well known and if pressure is too deep or too long sustained the resistance and tension that may be created can make the treatment counter-productive. It is possible to achieve deep, penetrating pressure, if it is variable in nature and not long held, without undue pain or discomfort. Thus a thinking, intuitive feel for the work is a prerequisite of successful application. Should trigger points be located, as indicated by the reproduction in a target area of an existing pain pattern, then sustained pressure is required for between ten seconds and two minutes. Even this sustained pressure should be slightly variable, i.e. deep pressure for ten seconds followed by a slight easing for a further ten seconds and so on, repeated until the reference pain diminishes or until the maximum time (two minutes) has elapsed. No more than this amount of manual pressure should be applied to a trigger point at any one session.

If, however, this has failed to minimize the referred pain it is often desirable to attempt to further ease the pain by applying ultrasound (pulsed) or a cold application, followed by stretching of the involved muscle, at the same session.

Once the right thumb has completed its series of transverse strokes across the long axis of the cervical musculature, the left hand, which has been resting on the patient's left shoulder, now comes into play. A series of strokes are applied upward from the left of the upper dorsal area towards the base of the skull. The fingers of the left hand rest (and act as a fulcrum) on the front of the shoulder area at the level of the medial aspect of the clavicle. The thumb tip should be angled to allow direct pressure to be exerted against the left lateral aspects of the upper dorsal and the lower cervical spinous processes as it glides cephalid. The subsequent strokes of the thumb should be in the same direction but slightly more laterally placed. The fingers should then be placed on the patient's head at about the temporo-occipital articulation. The left thumb then deals in the same way with the mid and upper cervical soft tissues, finishing with a lateral stroke or two across the insertions on the occiput itself.

In travelling from the nuchal line to the level of the cervico-dorsal junction and back again in a series of overlapping gliding movements, a number of possible trigger points will have been passed. The mid-point of the sterno-mastoid, at the level of the posterior angle of the jaw, can be a source of intense pain which may be felt above the temple in the ear region, below the angle of the jaw (see illustrations in Chapter 3). Similar triggers exist in the splenius capitus, trapzius, posterior cervical and other muscles of the area, all with different target areas. A degree of practice will soon allow these to be speedily located, identified and dealt with.

Posterior Reflex Centres Also in this area there occur the posterior reflex centres of the neuro-lymphatic type (Chapman's Reflexes), notably those connected with conjunctivitis, cerebellar congestion and ear, nose and throat problems of an inflammatory or congested type, from sinusitus to tonsillitis. Again it is suggested that due study is made of the illustrations in Chapter 4. Treatment of these points is via lightly sustained pressure.

Recall at this point that Gutstein (Chapter 2) found trigger areas in the cervical and upper dorsal region which profoundly affected such diverse conditions as menopausal symptoms, imbalance in skin secretions and excessive perspiration. He stressed the importance of the cervical region and the interscapular area. Among the more important *Tsubo* or acupressure points in the upper cervical area are: Gall Bladder 20, which lies bilaterally in a depression midway between the occipital protuberance and the mastoid at the base of the skull; Bladder 10, which lies bilaterally just lateral to the large bundle of muscular insertions at the occiput; and Triple Heater 17, which lies bilaterally in the depression between the lobe of ear and the mastoid process. These points, if sensitive, should receive a sustained or variable pressure as for the other trigger points. Their influence is felt in a variety of conditions relating to the head, such as migraine, neuralgia, cold symptoms, hyper- and hypo-tension, liver dysfunction etc.

Goodheart mentions levator scapulae 'weakness' as indicating digestive problems and recommends pressure techniques in the cervico-dorsal area and on the medial border of the scapula to help normalize this.

During the treatment special notice should be given to the origins and insertions of the muscles of the area. Where these bony landmarks are palpable by the thumb tip they should be treated by the slow, variably applied pressure technique. Indeed, all bony surfaces within reach of the probing digit should be searched for undue sensitivity and dysfunction. This left cervical area treatment should take no more than two minutes and, in the absence of dysfunction, can be comfortably and successfully dealt with in no more than 90 seconds. Indeed the entire basic spinal NMT treatment can usually be completed in ten to fifteen minutes.

Stanley Lief employed few specific manipulative techniques. His main concern was to attempt to normalize mobility and function (circulation, drainage, nerve function, etc.) and to this end his neuro-muscular treatment was often accompanied by no more than general rotary movements of the cervical and lumbar areas together with a degree of 'springing' or stretching of the dorsal region. Derision on the part of the 'specific' manipulators should be tempered by the fact that this general treatment approach (some would call it 'engine wiping') achieves phenomenal results in terms of improvement in general well being and the alleviation of many specific lesion patterns. Undoubtedly there are specific spinal and joint problems that require an individual approach, however, the correction of the supporting mechanism, via NMT on its own or together with general mobilizing techniques of manipulation, is able to frequently obviate the need for any more detailed technique. Indeed, specific adjusting, which pays no heed to the soft tissue component, is far more likely to fail (in the sense that symptoms speedily return) than the Lief method.

General Treatment Approach

Whichever hand is operating at any given time, the other hand can give assistance by means of gently rocking or stretching tissues to compliment the efforts of the treating hand. Following the treatment of the left side the same procedures are repeated on the right. As the operator changes side it is suggested that one hand maintains light contact with the patient. Indeed it is suggested that once treatment has commenced no breaks in contact be allowed. There is often a noticable increase in tension in the tissues of the patient if the series of strokes, stretching movements and pressure techniques etc. which make up NMT is interrupted by even a few seconds. A continuity of contact would seem, in itself, to be of therapeutic value, simply as a reassuring and calming measure.

Continuity of Contact

Once both left and right cervical areas have been treated the operator moves to the head of the plinth. Resting the tips of the fingers on the lower, lateral aspect of the neck the thumb tips are placed just lateral to the first dorsalspinal process. A degree of downward (towards the floor) pressure is applied via the thumbs which are then drawn cephalid alongside the lateral margins of the cervical spinous processes. This bilateral stroke culminates at the occiput where a lateral stretch or pull is introduced across the bunched fibres of the muscles inserting into the base of the skull.

The upward stroke should contain an element of pressure towards the spinous process so that the pad of the thumb is pressing downward (towards the floor) whilst the lateral thumb tip is directed towards the centre, attempting to contact the bony contours of the spine, all the time being drawn slowly cephalid to end at the occiput. This combination stroke is repeated two or three times. The fingertips which have been resting on the sterno-mastoid may also be employed at this stage to lift and stretch it posteriorly and laterally. The lateral stretch across the occipital protruberance may be likened to trying to break open a melon. The thumb tips dig deep into the medial fibres of the para-occipital bundle and an outward stretch is instituted, using the leverage of the arms, as though attempting to open out the occiput. The thumbs are then drawn laterally across the fibres of muscular insertion into the skull, in a series of strokes culminating at the occipito-parietal junction.

Figure 13b

Neuro-muscular Technique. Illustrating position of operator and lines of application.

The fingertips which act as a fulcrum to these movements rest on the mastoid area of the temporal bone. Several strokes are then performed by one thumb or the other running caudad directly over the spinous process from the base of the skull to the upper dorsal area. Pressure should be fairly strong and slow. In the same position the left thumb will now be placed on the right, lateral aspect of the first dorsal vertebra and a series of strokes are performed caudad and laterally as well as diagonally towards the scapula.

The fingers are splayed out ahead of the thumb in whichever direction it is travelling so that the force transmitted via the extended arm can be controlled. The fingers act as a fulcrum with the thumb tip being drawn across the palm towards the diagonally opposite point—the tip of the middle or little finger. The thumb should never lead the hand nor be solely 'digging' or pressing without the stabilizing and controlling action of the hand or fingertips also being in operation.

A series of strokes, shallow and then deep, is therefore applied from D1 to about D4 or 5 and outwards towards the scapula and along and across the upper trapezius fibres. The left hand treats the right side, and vice-versa with the non-operative hand resting on the neck or head. Weight transfer to the thumb is achieved by simply leaning forward. The treating arm and thumb should be relatively straight. A 'hooked' thumb in which all the work is done by the distal phalange will become extremely tired and will not achieve the degree of penetration possible via a fairly rigid thumb.

Some operators have hypermobile joints and it is difficult for them to maintain sustained pressure without the thumb giving way and bending back on itself. This is a problem which can only be overcome by attempting to build up the muscular strength of the hand or by using a variation of the above technique, e.g. a knuckle or even the elbow may be used to achieve deep pressure in very tense musculature.

Trapezius and Sterno-mastoid Muscles

Since it is difficult to apply pressure to the trapezius or sterno-mastoid muscles in such a way as to involve underlying bony structures it is necessary to lightly pinch or squeeze the more sensitive areas of dysfunction to assess trigger points and their related target areas of pain. By using the illustrations in Chapter 3 the location of the trigger points can be predicted and their presence rapidly established. When it is not possible to apply thumb pressure to such a point, a squeezing of the involved muscle area for from ten seconds to two minutes with varying pressure, will usually induce a diminution of the referred pain. Once this begins the pressure should be released. If no success is achieved by these means then chilling and stretching should be employed. Several strokes should then be applied directly over the spinous processes caudad to approximately the mid-dorsal area.

Left Side Treatment

The operator then moves to the patient's left side standing in the same manner as at the commencement of the treatment but at the level of the patient's waist. With the right hand now resting at the level of the lower dorsal spine the left thumb commences a series of strokes cephalid from the mid-dorsal area. Each stroke covers two or three spinal segments and runs immediately lateral to the spinous process so that the angle of pressure imparted via the medial tip of the thumb is roughly towards the contra-lateral nipple. Again, light and deep strokes are employed and a degree of overlap is allowed on successive strokes.

In this way the first two strokes might run from D8 to D5 followed by two strokes (one light, one deeper) from D6 to D3 and finally two strokes from D4 to D1. Deeper and more sustained pressure should be exerted upon discovering marked congestion or resistance to the gliding, probing thumb. In the dorsal area a second line of upward strokes may be employed to include the spinal border of the scapula as well as one or two searching lateral probes along the inferior spine of the scapula and across the musculature inferior to and inserting into the scapula.

Right Side Treatment

Treatment of the right side may be carried out without necessarily changing position, other than to lean across the patient. However, the shorter practitioner should change sides so that, standing half-facing the head of the patient, the right thumb can perform the strokes discussed above. Apart from trigger points in the lower trapezius fibres others may be sought in levator scapulae, supra and infra spinatus, and subscapularis. Remember that the connective tissue zones affecting the arm, stomach, heart, liver and gall bladder are apparent in the region now being treated. Neuro-lymphatic reflexes relating to the arm, thyroid,

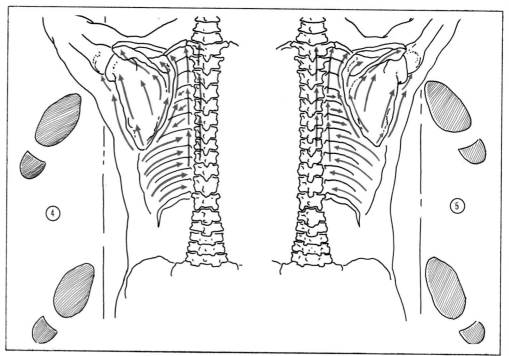

Figure 13c

Neuro-muscular Technique. Illustrating position of operator and lines of application.

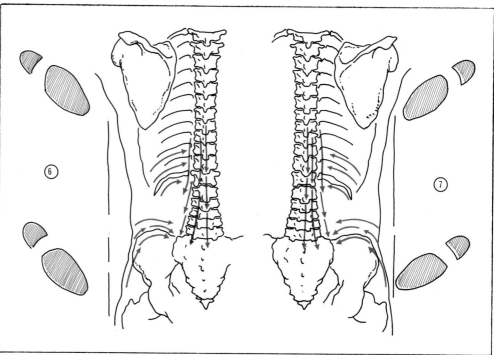

Figure 13d

Neuro-muscular Technique. Illustrating position of operator and lines of application.

lungs, throat and heart occur in the upper dorsal spine including the scapular area.

The intercostal spaces are a rich site of dysfunction. The thumb tip or a fingertip should be run along both surfaces of the rib margin as well as in the intercostal space itself. In this way the fibres of the small muscles involved will be adequately treated. If there is overapproximation of the ribs then a simple stroke along the space may be all that is possible until a degree of normalization has taken place. These intercostal areas are extremely sensitive and care must be taken not to distress the patient.

The practitioner now half turns so that instead of facing the patient's head he faces the patient's feet. The pattern of strokes is now carried out on the patient's left side by the operator's right hand. A series starting from D8 to D11 followed by D11 to L1, and then L1 to L4 is carried out as before. Two or more gliding strokes with the pressure downwards but angled so that the medial aspect of the thumb is in contact with the lateral margin of the spinous process, are performed at each level.   **Change of Position**

The intercostal areas are again treated as described above. The operator steps away from the plinth and glides the thumb along the superior iliac spine from just above the hip to the sacro-iliac joint. Several such strokes may be applied into the heavy musculature above the crest of ilium. The right side application requires the operator to change sides so that facing the patient's waist and half-turned towards the feet, the left hand can deal with the lower dorsal and upper lumbar area and the iliac crest in the manner described above. One or two strokes should then be applied running caudad over the tips of the spinous processes from the mid-dorsal area to the sacrum.

The area we have been describing contains a veritable network of reflex areas and points. The *Tsubo* or acupressure points lying symmetrically on either side of the spine and along the midline have great reflex importance. The so-called 'Bladder' points lie in two lines running parallel with the spine, one level with the medial border of the scapula and the other midway between it and the lateral border of the spinous processes.

Goodheart's work suggests that rhomboid weakness indicates liver problems and that pressure on C7 spinous process and a point on the right of the interspace between the fifth and sixth dorsal spinous process assists its normalization. Latissimus dorsi weakness apparently indicates pancreatic dysfunction. Lateral to seventh and eighth dorsal interspace is the posterior pressure reflex to normalize this. These and other reflexes would appear to derive from Chapman's Reflex theories and are deserving of further study.

In general terms, dysfunction of the erector spinae group of muscles between sixth and twelfth dorsal indicates liver involvement. Similarly fourth, fifth and sixth dorsal area congestion or sensitivity usually involves stomach reflexes and gastric disturbance, whereas D12 and L2 indicates possible kidney dysfunction.

The next treatment position requires the operator to stand at the level of the patient's left hip, half-facing the head of the couch. The left hand and thumb   **Left Hip Position**

Figure 14

Operator using Neuro-muscular Technique. Note position of feet; straight right arm; right hand position; thumb position. See drawing No. 6 on page 102.

describe a series of cephalid strokes from the sacral apex towards the sacro-iliac area and then laterally along the superior and inferior margins of the iliac crest to the insertion of the tensor fascia lata at the anterior, superior iliac spine. A further series of short strokes of the thumb upwards and laterally in the lumbar area are best described as attempting to stretch and open out from the spine the muscles of the area, notably the sacro-spinal group.

Having treated both left and right sides of the lumbar spine as above the operator uses a series of two-handed gliding manoeuvres in which the hands are spread over the upper gluteal area laterally, the thumb tips are placed at the level of the second sacral foramen with a downward (towards the floor) pressure; they glide cephalid and slowly laterally to pass over and through the fibres of the sacro-iliac joint. This is repeated several times.

Still standing on the left, the operator leans across the patient's upper thigh and engages his right thumb onto the ischial tuberosity. A series of gliding movements are carried out from that point laterally to the hip and caudad towards the gluteal fold. A further series of strokes, always applying deep, probing, but variable pressure is then carried out from the sacral border across the gluteal area to the hip margins. The fingertips during these strokes are splayed out so that they can guide and balance the hand and thumb movement. In these deep muscles the line of the thumb's direction is more towards the tip of the index finger or middle finger rather than to the little fingertip, as it was in the cervical area. In deep, tense gluteal muscle the thumb can be inadequate to the task of prolonged pressure techniques and the elbow may be used to sustain deep pressure for minutes at a time. Care should be taken, however, as the degree of pressure possible by this means is enormous and tissue damage and bruising can result from its careless employment.

Figure 13e

Neuro-muscular Technique. Illustrating position of operator and lines of application.

The trigger points that may be sought for in the lower lumbar and gluteal areas include those in the following muscle groups: iliocostal, multifidus, longissimus, gluteus medius and gluteus minimus. The connective tissue zones that may be involved include those that involve arterial and venous disturbance to the legs, constipation, liver, gall bladder, heart and bladder.

The neuro-lymphatic reflexes include those that involve the following areas and conditions: the appendix, haemorrhoids, female generative organs, vasiculitis, sciatic nerve, abdominal tension and constipation, prostate, colitis, kidneys, adrenal glands, digestive system, pancreas, liver, spleen and gall bladder.

Having treated the low lumbar area and the gluteals the operator might (if the low back is a problem area) include a series of strokes across the fibres of the tensor fascia lata from the hip area to the lateral knee area. The tensor fascia lata contains neuro-lymphatic reflexes to the groin glands, the broad ligaments, spastic constipation and colitis, prostate etc.

Completion of Treatment

This completes the basic spinal NMT treatment apart from any manipulative procedures that might be indicated or thought desirable. Boris Chaitow completes the spinal treatment by standing at the head of the plinth leaning over the patient's upper dorsal area, the palms of both hands totally in contact with the upper lumbar region so that the thenar eminence is resting on the paraspinal musculature and the fingers pointing laterally. The heel of the hand imparts the main contact laterally. A series of gliding strokes is performed with the hands rhythmically alternating with each other so that as the right hand strokes downwards to end its movement on the gluteals the left is being brought back to the lower dorsal area. After it descends the right hand comes back to the start. In this way a series of ten to twenty deep rhythmic strokes are carried out in order to stimulate local circulation and drainage as well as to further relax the patient who may well have tensed during the treatment of the lumbar and gluteal areas.

As stated previously, the basic treatment should take no more than fifteen minutes. The patient should have a sense of release from tension and of well being. This may last for some days. Many feel a sense of tiredness and a great desire to sleep, this should be encouraged. Pain may result in those areas that have borne the main brunt of the pressure techniques. This should be explained to the patient who should be encouraged to note any changes in his condition and to report these at the subsequent visit. The frequency of application of NMT will vary with the condition. In chronic conditions one or two treatments weekly are as much as is ever required. This can be maintained until progress dictates that the interval be lengthened. In acute conditions treatment may be much more frequent, daily if possible until ease is achieved. Of necessity this must depend upon what other modalities are employed.

A simple, precise technique for the alleviation of local and reflex pain, the normalizing and balancing of muscular tone, the restoration of functional harmony and the release of physical and psychic tension is available to all with the patience and intelligence to know what their hands are feeling and to employ the methods developed by Stanley Lief and his followers.

Chapter 6

Basic Abdominal Technique

In treating the abdominal and related areas our attention should focus on specific junctional tissues. These comprise the central tendon and the lateral aspect of the rectal muscle sheaths, the insertion of the recti muscles and external oblique muscles into the ribs, the xiphisternal ligament as well as the lower insertions of the internal and external oblique muscles. The intercostal areas from fifth to twelfth ribs are equally important.

Specific general areas are worthy of consideration in treating conditions affecting particular organs or functions.

Liver dysfunction and portal circulatory dysfunction would call for special attention to the right side intercostal musculature from fifth to twelfth ribs. Especially important are the various muscular insertions into all these ribs.

Gall bladder dysfunction involves the above areas with extra attention to the area on the costal margin, roughly midway between the xiphisternal notch and the lateral rib margins.

Spleen function may be stimulated by attention to the intercostal spaces between the seventh and twelfth ribs on the left side.

Digestive disorders in general will benefit from NMT applied to the central tendon between the recti and directly to the rectal sheaths.

Stomach pain is treated via its reflex area to the left of the xiphisternal notch and to the tendon and rectal sheaths.

Colonic problems and ovarian dysfunction will benefit from reflex NMT application to both iliac fossae as well as to the midline structures.

Dysfunction of the kidneys, ureters and bladder require attention to the inguinal borders of the internal and external oblique insertions, the suprapubic insertions of the recti, the overlying muscles and sheaths of the area and the internal aspects of the upper thigh.

In pelvic congestion relating to gynaecological dysfunction NMT should be applied to the hypogastrium and both iliac fossae. This relieves congestion and stimulates pelvic circulation.

Ileitis and other functional disturbances of the transverse colon and small intestine benefit from NMT applied to the umbilical area.

Prostatic dysfunction will benefit from NMT to the central hypogastric region. Internal drainage massage of the prostate should also be considered.

Gutstein's myodysneuric points.

Figure 15a

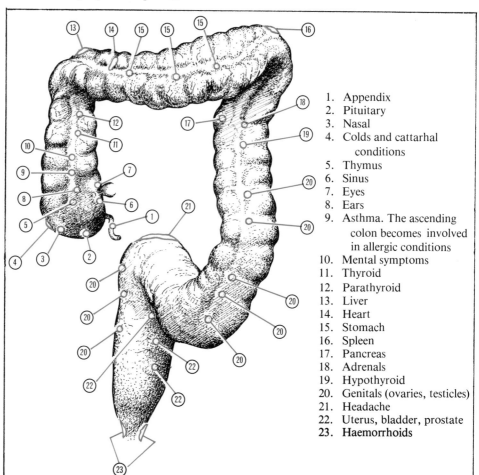

1. Appendix
2. Pituitary
3. Nasal
4. Colds and cattarhal conditions
5. Thymus
6. Sinus
7. Eyes
8. Ears
9. Asthma. The ascending colon becomes involved in allergic conditions
10. Mental symptoms
11. Thyroid
12. Parathyroid
13. Liver
14. Heart
15. Stomach
16. Spleen
17. Pancreas
18. Adrenals
19. Hypothyroid
20. Genitals (ovaries, testicles)
21. Headache
22. Uterus, bladder, prostate
23. **Haemorrhoids**

Fielder's reflex areas of the large intestine.

Figure 15b

The above brief indications should be considered in conjunction with other reflex systems and points (see below) as well as to the appropriate spinal areas which would also receive NMT treatment.

Abdominal Reflex Areas

Gutstein[1] has noted trigger areas in the sternal, parasternal and epigastric regions and the upper portions of the rectus, all relating to varying degrees of retro-peristalsis. He also noted that colonic dysfunction related to triggers in the mid and lower rectus muscle. These were all predominantly left-sided. Other symptoms which improved or disappeared with the obliteration of these triggers include excessive appetite, poor appetite, flatulence, nervous vomiting, nervous diarrhoea etc. The triggers were always tender spots, easily found by the palpation and situated mainly in the upper, mid and lower portions of the recti muscles, over the lower portion of the sternum and the epigastrium including the xyphoid process and the parasternal regions. The parasternal region corresponds to the insertions of the rectus muscle into the fifth, sixth and seventh ribs *(see Figure 15a)*.

Fielder[2] described a number of reflexes occurring on the large bowel itself. These could be localized by deep palpation and treated by specific release techniques *(see Figure 15b)*.

These reflexes palpate as areas of tenderness and may include a degree of swelling and congestion resulting from adhesions, spasticity, diverticuli, chemical or bacterial irritation etc.

In considering the reflexes available in the thoracic and abdominal regions the neuro-lymphatic points of Chapman are also worthy of close attention. To what extent Gutstein's myodysneuric points are interchangeable with Chapman's reflexes or Fielder's reflexes or other systems of reflex study (e.g. acupuncture or Tsubo points and Travell's triggers) and to what extent these involve Mackenzie's work *(see Figure 3)* is a matter for further research. *Suffice it to say that within the soft tissue structures of this region there abound palpable, sensitive, discrete areas of dysfunction which, on a local basis, interfere with or modify functional integrity to a greater or lesser degree, and reflexly are capable of massive interference with normal physiological function on a neural, circulatory and lymphatic level, to the extent of producing or mimicking serious pathological conditions.* Since these areas of dysfunction will often yield to simple, soft tissue manipulative techniques, which are incorporated into Lief's NMT, the value of these techniques becomes apparent.

Mackenzie[3] and others demonstrated a clear relationship between the abdominal wall and the viscera. This and other reflex patterns provide the rationale for NMT application to the abdominal and sternal regions. These reflex patterns vary in individual cases but it is clear that the majority of the organs are able to protect themselves by producing contraction, spasm and hyperaesthesia of the overlying, reflexly related muscle wall, the myotome. This is often augmented by hyperaesthesia of the overlying skin as well, the dermatome. These reflexes are via the autonomic reflex pathways *(see Figure 3)*.

In treating the abdominal and thoracic regions the patient should be supine with the head supported by a medium-sized pillow and the knees flexed, either

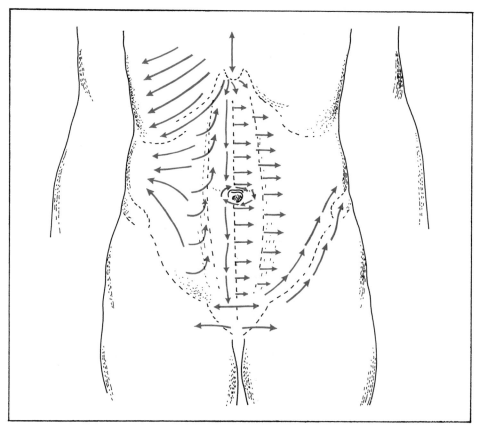

Figure 16

Neuro-muscular general abdominal technique. Lines of application.

with a bolster under them or drawn right up so that the feet approximate the buttocks. Generous application of lubricant should be made to the area being treated.

Intercostal The operator positions himself so that he is level with the patient's waist and a
Treatment series of strokes are applied with the tip of the thumb along the course of the intercostal spaces from the sternum, laterally. It is important that the insertions of the internal and external muscles receive attention. The margins of the ribs, both inferior and superior aspects, should receive firm gliding pressure from the distal phalanx of the thumb or middle finger. If there is too little space to allow such a degree of differentiated pressure then a simple stroke along the available intercostal space suffices.

The intercostals from the fifth rib to the costal margin are given a series of two or three deep, slow-moving, gliding, sensitive strokes on each side with special reference to points of particular congestion or sensitivity. These areas may benefit from thirty to sixty seconds of sustained or variable pressure techniques. These points will not bear heavy pressure techniques such as may be required in more heavily muscled regions and caution is called for. The operator should bear in mind the various reflex patterns in the region. Gentle probing on the sternum itself may elicit sensitivity in the rudimentary sternalis muscle. If this is found to be sensitive then variable pressure treatment should be applied.

It is not necessary for the operator to change sides during the treatment of the intercostals unless it is found to be more comfortable to do so.

The operator should be facing the patient and be half-turned towards the head with legs apart for an even distribution of weight and with knees flexed to facilitate the transfer of pressure through the arms. Since many of the manoeuvres in the intercostal area and on the abdomen itself involve finger and thumb movements of a lighter nature than those applied through the heavy spinal musculature the elbows need not be kept so straight.

However, when deep pressure is called for, and especially when this is applied via the thumb, the same criterion of weight transference from the shoulder through the thumb applies and the straightish arm is then an advantage for the economic and efficient use of energy.

Having treated the intercostal musculature and connective tissue and used pressure techniques to deal with any trigger points that have been elicited, the operator, using either a deep thumb pressure or a contact with the pads of the fingertips, applies a series of short strokes in a combination of oblique lateral and inferior directions from the xyphoid process.

Rectal Sheath

This is followed by the same contact in a series of deep slow strokes along and under the costal margins. A series of short strokes with fairly deep but not painful pressure is then applied by the thumb, from the midline up to the lateral rectal sheath. This series of strokes starts just inferior to the xyphoid and concludes at the pubic promontory. This series may be repeated on each side several times depending upon the degree of tension, congestion and sensitivity.

A similar pattern of treatment is followed across the lateral border of the rectal sheath. A series of short, deep, slow-moving thumb strokes being applied from just inferior to the costal margin of the rectal sheath until the inguinal ligament is reached. Both sides are treated in this way.

A series of similar strokes is then applied on the one side and then the other laterally from the lateral border of the rectal sheath. These strokes follow the contour of the trunk so that the upper strokes travel in a slightly inferior curve whilst passing laterally and the lower strokes have a superior inclination, as the hand passes laterally. A total of five or six strokes would be adequate to complete these movements and this could be repeated before performing the same movements on the opposite side.

In treating the side on which the operator is standing it may be more comfortable to apply the therapeutic stroke via the flexed finger tips which are drawn towards the operator, or the usual thumb stroke may be used. In treating the opposite side, thumb pressure can more easily be applied, as in spinal technique, with the fingers acting as a fulcrum and the thumb gliding towards them in a series of two- or three-inch long strokes. The sensing of contracted, gangliform areas of dysfunction is more difficult in abdominal work and requires great sensitivity of touch and concentration on the part of the operator.

Symphysis Pubis   Attention should be given to the insertions into, and the soft tissue component of, the pubic bones and the symphysis pubis. A deep but not painful stroke, employing the pad of the thumb, should be applied to the superior aspect of the pubic crest. This should start at the symphysis pubis and move laterally, first in one direction and, after repeating it once or twice, then the other. A similar series, starting at the centre and moving laterally, should then be applied over the anterior aspect of the pubic bone. Great care should be taken not to use undue pressure as the area is sensitive at the best of times and may be acutely so if there is dysfunction associated with the insertions into these structures. A series of deep slow movements is then performed, via the thumb, along the superior and inferior aspects of the inguinal ligament, starting at the pubic bone and running up to and beyond the iliac crest.

The thumbs or fingertips may then be insinuated beneath the lateral rectus border at its lower margins and deep pressure applied towards the midline. The hand or thumb should then slowly move cephalid in short stages whilst maintaining this medial pressure. This lifts the connective tissue from its underlying attachments and helps to normalize localized contractures and fibrous infiltrations.

Umbilicus   A series of strokes should then be applied around the umbilicus. Using thumb or flexed fingertips a number of movements of a stretching nature should be performed in which the non-treating hand stabilizes the tissue at the start of the stroke which firstly runs from approximately one inch superior and lateral to the umbilicus on the right side to the same level on the left side. The non-treating hand then stabilizes the tissues at this end point of the stroke and a further stretching and probing stroke is applied inferiorly to a point about one inch inferior and lateral to the umbilicus on the left side. This area is then stabilized and the stroke is applied to a similar point on the right.

The circle is completed by a further stroke upwards to end at the point at which the series began. This series of movements should have a rhythmical pattern so that as the treating hand reaches the end of its stroke the non-treating hand comes to that point and replaces the contact as a stabilizing pressure whilst the treating hand begins its next movement. A series of three or four such circuits of the umbilicus is performed.

Additional strokes may be applied along the midline and the sheaths of the recti muscles from the costal margins downwards. A soothing culmination to the foregoing ten to fifteen minutes may be applied by a circular clockwise series of movements in which the palm of one hand and the heel of the other alternately circle the whole abdominal area. Thus, with the operator standing to the right of the patient, the palm and fingers of the left hand stroke deeply but gently down the left abdominal structures and then across the lower abdomen towards the operator where, using the heel and palm, the right hand takes over the stroke and proceeds up the right side to the costal margin. As this point it changes direction to run across the upper abdomen where the left hand takes over to the repeat this pattern several times.

Specific release techniques *(see page 71)* may be applied during or after this general treatment. Such abdominal treatment can be repeated several times weekly if indicated but normally once a week is adequate until normality is achieved. In chronic conditions of abdominal or pelvic dysfunction the foregoing approach, together with specific release movements and appropriate spinal treatment will have a profound effect on function in the area. With an improvement in circulation and drainage and a reduction in tensions, contractions and reflex activities, the homeostatic mechanisms of the body will ensure an overall increase in energy and an improvement in the mechanical integrity and biochemical activity of the individual with a consequent lifting of the level of health. Many chronic dysfunctions and problems will simply disappear after a series of NMT abdominal techniques.

[1] Gutstein, R., 'The Role of Abdominal Fibrositis in Functional Indigestion', *Mississippi Valley Medical Journal* (1944), pp. 66-114.
[2] Fielder and Pyott, *The Science and Art of Manipulative Surgery* (American Institute of Manipulative Surgery Inc., 1955).
[3] Mackenzie, Sir James, *Symptoms and Their Interpretation* (London, 1909).

Chapter 7

Postural Considerations

Posture represents the sum of the mechanical efficiency of the body. It may be read as a book to assess the integrity, potential and, to some extent, the history of the individual.

The ideal posture is one in which the different segments of the body, the head, neck, chest, and abdomen are balanced vertically one upon the other so that the weight is borne mainly by the bony framework with a minimum of effort and strain on muscles and ligaments.

For such posture to be maintained special postural muscles must be in a state of constant activity. These have a special physiological property called 'postural activity'. These muscles include the sacrospinalis, glutei, quadriceps, sartorius and, to some extent, the calf muscles.

Correct posture is one in which the head is centred over the pelvis, the face directed forward, and the shoulder girdle approximately on the same plane as the pelvis.

The individual with poor posture may be described as one whose head is carried forward, whose scapulae are held in abduction, giving the shoulders a rounded appearance, whose dorsal curve is increased, and whose chest is flattened. Lordosis and prominence of the anterior abdominal wall below the level of the umbilicus is accompanied by an anterior tilt of the pelvis, the knees being slightly flexed.

Even the slightest alteration in the normal balance of the various spinal segments is accompanied by some degree of soft tissue change. Poor posture may not produce immediate pathological symptoms but must be considered as a potential cause of trouble later.

Structure and Function Relationship

The inter-relationship between structure and function is total. The way the human machine is used and misused will greatly influence its structures. The structural changes engendered by postural and other, perhaps traumatic, insults will determine its ability to function mechanically. The soft tissues are the supporting structures which connect, bind, support and which provide stability and allow free motion to the articulations of the body.

The ability to contract and relax are the major attributes of most soft tissues.

As a result of injury, disease or wrong use these soft tissues can undergo changes which include shortening, thickening, calcification and erosion. Changes in tension within fascial and connective tissue will occur depending upon the stresses imposed upon it by postural and other activities. This will result in reinforcement, shortening and thickening of these tissues. Excessive thickening can occur and this will accompany shortening, restriction of normal motion and probably alteration of positional integrity.

Postural defects can be shown to produce an accumulation of strain in the soft tissues (muscles, fascia, articular structures etc.) which predisposes towards dysfunction, pain and tenderness, especially in areas of bony attachment, areas of calcification and in areas where stress forces converge. When the deep fascia is subject to stress forces the collagenous fibres will be deposited which may create stress bands along the lines of force. Excessive tensions exerted by fascia and muscles on an area of articular dysfunction may make manipulative correction difficult or impossible.

The position of the bony framework is determined by the soft tissues which invest, support, bind and move it. Faulty tensions in these soft tissues will lead to abnormalities in the skeletal structure and therefore of its function, and possibly of the organs and functions (blood vessels etc.) which are also supported by connective, fascial tissue and muscle. Not only is the soft tissue subject to gravitational stress but also to a battery of postural and occupational stresses overlaid with the normal contraction that comes with age.

Postural Fascia

There are specializations of fascia, such as plantar, iliotibial, gluteal, lumbodorsal, cervical and cranial which stabilize and permit maintenance of the upright posture. Some of the fascial specializations of the body are referred to as 'postural fascia' because they have a special postural function and are among the first to show changes in the presence of postural defects. They assist in producing the necessary stabilization and, at the same time, permit motion initiated by muscular activity. Fascia is supplied with sensory nerves and many of its specializations previously mentioned are characterized by stress or tension bands of varying thickness.

Wherever the deep fascia is subjected to tension, it is reinforced in some way; for example, it may be further strengthened by deposition of paraneural bundles of collagenous fibres so that they form a definite aponeurosis. Dr Leon Page[1] points out:

> The cervical visceral fascia extends from the base of the skull to the mediastinum and forms compartments enclosing the oesophagus, trachea, carotid vessels and provides support for the pharynx, larynx and thyroid gland. There is a direct continuity of fascia from the apex of the diaphragm to the base of the skull. Extending through the fibrous pericardium upward through the deep cervical fascia the continuity extends not only to the outer surface of the sphenoid, occipital, and temporal bones but proceeds further through the foramina in the base of the skull around the vessels and nerves to joint the dura.

Thus it can be seen that the respiratory movements or the positions of the head and neck could have an influence upon the intracranial structures purely through continuity of fascia as well as upon the thoracic visceral and vascular structures.

This provides part of the rationale behind cranial manipulative techniques. At birth much of the connective tissue is loose and poorly defined. Abnormal tensions during development may result from trauma, faulty nutrition, wrong use etc. and encourage posture bands to become fixed in states of unequal tension. This may result in shortening and thickening of fascia and of osseous structures into irregular patterns. Structural imbalance increases the load on postural muscles and fascia with consequent reinforcement of these abnormal states.

It should be recalled that in the human the degree of hip extension required for the upright posture is dependent on the hamstring and gluteus maximus muscles which also initiate knee joint extension together with the quadriceps femoris. The tensor fascia lata provides the opposing force for the hypertensors. These all deserve attention in diagnostic and therapeutic terms.

Low Back Pain   In a major study of posture Lawrence Jones M.D., analysed 500 cases of chronic low back pain. These cases included only those that had as their chief complaint chronic low back pain of at least ninety days continuous duration and which were intractable to previous treatment. Comparative study showed that this condition is a clinical rarity prior to the age of twenty. The main age for onset lies between thirty and sixty years of age indicating that 'the loss of elasticity of soft tissues and other changes that accompany age progression play a major role in bringing to the surface previously latent conditions'.

It is significant that if individuals have not developed low back pain before the age of sixty, susceptibility to this symptom almost disappears (apart from symptoms of organic origin).

Over 80 per cent of the cases in this study had had their symptoms for over five years. A generalized pattern of allied symptoms, indicated an essential unity of postural involvement. These allied symptoms include fatigue, general leg ache, sciatica and upper nerve root involvement. Jones considers generalized fatigue such a common accompaniment of chronic low back pain as to be considered as an outstanding diagnostic symptom of a postural etiology.

Jones' solution to the problem is by correction of the feet by means of a fixed postural shoe. He claims that 15 per cent of chronic cases are substantially relieved within ten days and over 40 per cent within a month. In their classic *Essentials of Body Mechanics* Goldthwait et al show unequivocally the connection between the postural aspect and generalized ill health. To quote on just one aspect of this:

It has been shown that the main factors which determine the maintenance of the abdominal viscera in position are the diaphragm and abdominal muscles, both of which are relaxed and cease to support in faulty posture. The disturbances of circulation from a low diaphragm and ptosis may give rise to chronic passive congestion in one or all of the organs of the abdomen and pelvis, since the local as well as general venous drainage may be impeded by the failure of the diaphragmatic pump to do its full work in the drooped body. Furthermore, the drag of these congested organs on their nerve supply, as well as the pressure on the sympathetic ganglia and plexuses, probably causes many irregularities in their function, varying from partial paralysis to overstimulation. All these organs receive fibres from both the vagus and sympathetic systems, either one of which may be disturbed. It is probable that one or all of these factors are active at various times in both the stocky and the slender anatomic types, and are responsible for many functional digestive disturbances. These disturbances, if continued long enough may lead to diseases in later life. Faulty body mechanics in early life, then, becomes a vital factor in the production of the vicious cycle of chronic diseases and presents the chief point of attack in its prevention. . . . In this upright position, as one becomes older, the tendency is for the abdomen to relax and sag more and more, allowing a ptosic condition of the abdominal and pelvic organs unless the supporting lower abdominal muscles are taught to contract properly. As the abdomen relaxes, there is a great tendency toward a drooped chest, with a narrowed rib angle, forward shoulders, prominent shoulder blades, a forward position of the head, and probably pronated feet. When the human machine is out of balance, physiologic function cannot be perfect; muscles and ligaments are in an abnormal state of tension and strain. A well-poised body means a machine working perfectly, with the least amount of muscular effort, and therefore better health and strength for daily life.

Muscle Testing

In their study of posture Drs Kendall, Kendall and Boynton[3] have indicated that there exists a simple method of testing certain muscle groups in a postural context. Having repeatedly performed complete muscle tests on normal subjects they found certain groups that tended to show weakness in various particular postural or alignment problems. These muscles therefore represent the essential ones to be tested to assess the initial postural condition and to monitor progress.

It is not clear whether the postural faults precede or result from the muscle group weakness. Whenever muscle weakness exists some particular movement or degree of stability will be impaired. Tests as described are specific to the particular muscle. Where muscles that move the extremities are concerned the patient is required to hold the part in a specific position against the pull of gravity and against the maximum pressure exerted by the examiner.

In the case of small joints such as toes, gravity will play no part. A muscle that maintains its anti-gravity position against the operators pressure is graded as 100 per cent. If the muscle holds its antigravity test position against medium pressure then an 80-90 per cent grade is given. A 50 per cent mark indicates that only the antigravity position is held but that no added pressure is exerted on the part of the operator. Less than 50 per cent indicates a very weak muscle and probably a degree of pathology outside the scope of normal manual therapy. In the case of the anterior trunk muscles gravity alone is used.

Pressure should always be applied gradually by the operator as even a strong muscle will give way to suddenly applied pressure.

If there exists a joint immobility which restricts the range of the part so that the test canot be fully performed then the test should be carried out through the range that does exist.

Test for 'Lower' Abdominal Muscles

A person with 100 per cent 'lower' abdominal muscles is able to maintain the pelvis in a position of posterior tilt with the back flat while raising both legs from the table. The hands are placed behind the head. A narrowing of the costal angle indicates that the obliquus externus is contracting.

If the subject is unable to intitiate leg-raising without allowing the back to arch, the legs are brought (with assistance) to a nearly vertical position and the subject is asked to hold the back flat while slowly lowering the legs. The angle between the legs and the table when the back just begins to arch off the table is used to determine the muscle strength grade. If the angle is about 80° the grade is 50 per cent; if it is about 60° the grade if 60 per cent; if about 40° the grade is 80 per cent.

When the 'lower' abdominal muscle test is given to patients with back pain an effort is made to avoid strain on the back. The attempt to do double leg-raising is omitted and the test is done by checking for pelvic tilt during leg-lowering, as described above. Also in such cases, the arms are usually crossed on the chest instead of being placed under the head.

It will be noted that the rectus abdominis is one of the muscles primarily concerned in both the 'upper' and 'lower' abdominal tests. This does not mean that the action is confined to the upper and lower aspects of the rectus respectively. The terms 'upper' and 'lower' refer not to location of the muscles, but to the section of the trunk which is chiefly involved in the movement.

The 100 per cent standard for lower abdominal muscles is primarily a standard for adult males. For other individuals normal strength according to age may be considered as follows: infants, test not used; aged 4-12 years, 60 per cent to 70 per cent; aged 12 years to adults, 70 per cent to 80 per cent; adult women, 80 per cent.

The tests for strength of 'upper' and 'lower' abdominal muscles are important in all routine postural examinations.

Trunk-raising Test of 'Upper' Abdominal Muscles The starting position is supine with the hands clasped behind the head and the pelvis tilted backward to flatten the low back against the table. The subject should flex the trunk without jerking, raising first his head and then his shoulders. Through this arc, his feet should not come up from the table, but neither should they be held down by the operator. The change in the costal angle during the performance of abdominal tests indicates which of the oblique muscles is acting.

The second movement is flexion of the trunk on the thighs by the hip flexors. At this stage of the movement the legs may be held down if the weight of the legs does not counterbalance the weight of the trunk. If the hands are behind the head during the successful performance of the test a grade of 100 per cent can be given. A grade of 80 per cent is given if the movement can only be completed with the arms folded across the chest. For a 60 per cent result the arms would be extended diagonally forward during the movement. For a 50 per cent result the same arm position is used as for the 60 per cent but only the neck is capable of being raised by the patient, and not the shoulders.

If the subject with normal back flexibility is unable to perform to a grade of 50 per cent then the muscles are graded 'weak'. If the back muscles are very tight it must be determined whether abdominal weakness or back tightness has prevented completion of the test movement.

Patient supine, hands clasped behind the head. The examiner places the trunk in the exact test position of flexion and rotation, to an angle of 45° from the surface, and asks the subject to hold that position. If the strength of the muscles is 100 per cent the trunk will not drop or shift out of position. When the trunk is rotated forward on the right, the diagonal fibres of the right external and left internal oblique muscles are chiefly used. If the left side is rotated forward the left external and right internal oblique muscles are used.

Trunk-raising Test of Oblique Abdominal Muscles

The legs must be stabilized by an assistant during the performance of this test, and hip flexor strength must be adequate to stabilize the pelvis in this test position. For an 80 per cent test result the arms are folded on the chest and the shoulders are held only a few inches above the table. For a 60 per cent test result the arms are extended forward and the lower shoulder is barely lifted from the table. A 50 per cent result does not involve raising the trunk. With the examiner giving moderate resistance against a diagonally downward pull of the subject's arm, the cross-sectional pull of the oblique abdominal muscles should be very firm on palpation and should pull the costal margin toward the opposite iliac crest. The test may also be done by applying pressure against the thigh with the leg in about 60° hip flexion. The obliques should then pull the iliac crest toward the opposite costal margin. The test of the oblique abdominal muscles is most important in case of scoliosis.

The movement starts with the patient lying on his side, The upper arm is held along the side of his body. The lower arm is folded across the chest and the hand rests on the upper shoulder. Pillows are placed on top of and between the legs to prevent the discomfort of one leg pressing on the other as the operator stabilizes them by downward pressure. The subject raises the trunk by lifting first the head and then the shoulders sideways. There should be no rotation of the trunk. As the movement progresses, the upper side of the pelvis tilts downward a little to accommodate for the change in pelvic position. The examiner, in his effort to stabilize the legs, must not prevent the adjustment.

Test of Lateral Trunk Flexors

The ability to do this test movement correctly depends upon having a full range of motion in lateral trunk flexion as well as upon having adequate strength. The lateral trunk flexors are graded 100 per cent if the costal margin can be brought close to the iliac crest. If the lower shoulder is raised about four inches (10cm) from the table the muscle grade is 80 per cent. If the shoulder is raised only one to three inches (2.5-7.5cm) from the table the grade is 50 to 60 per cent. If the trunk fails to move through the full arc of motion the examiner must determine whether the primary reason is weakness of the muscles being tested or tightness of their opponents. The tests for strength of lateral trunk flexors are important in cases of lateral pelvic tilt and scoliosis.

Patient should be prone, with fists clenched and resting on the buttocks. Legs are stabilized by the operator whilst the patient lifts the head and thorax from the table. If the subject can hold this position against maximum pressure exerted downward on the upper dorsal spine by the examiner, the grade is 100 per cent. If the position is held against slight pressure the grade is 80 per cent. If the subject almost completes the full movement the grade is 60 per cent. If he raises high

Test of Back Extensor Muscles

enough to lift the lower end of the sternum from the table the grade is 50 per cent.

While exerting pressure on the upper back with one hand for the 100 per cent and 80 per cent tests, the examiner continues to stabilize the lower legs with the other hand.

The low back extensors are seldom weak in cases of typical faulty posture. However, since the erector spinae muscles are the most important of all the trunk muscles, it is necessary to detect weakness when it exists. For this reason, and because the routine examination of back extensors will dispel the mistaken idea that most painful low backs are 'weak' this test is included in the group of postural cases.

Test for Serratus Anterior
The serratus anterior holds the scapula close to the rib cage and rotates the inferior angle of the scapula forward. The sitting position is one of several which may be used for testing this muscle. The arm is placed in about 120° flexion and the examiner exerts downward pressure on the upper arm and backward pressure on the medial border of the scapula with the other hand. If the serratus anterior is weak the inferior angle of the scapula will rotate medially and the whole vertebral border of the scapula will stand out from the rib cage; the subject will be unable to hold the test position because of lack of adequate scapular stabilization.

Tests for strength of the serratus anterior should be done in cases of faulty scapular position, or in cases of pain in the area of the rhomboids since the latter may shorten and be painful in cases of serratus weakness.

Test of the Psoas Major
The subject is in a supine position. The examiner places the leg to be tested in a position of hip flexion, slight abduction and slight external rotation, and asks the subject to hold that position while he presses downward and slightly outward on the lower leg. The examiner stabilizes the opposite hip. The test for psoas major is of particular importance in cases of anterior deviation of the pelvis, lumbar kyphosis, or lumbar scoliosis. Weakness tends to be bilateral in cases of lumbar kyphosis, and unilateral in cases of lumbar scoliosis.

Test of Gluteus Medius (Posterior Part)
The subject lies on his side with the lower leg flexed at the hip and knee. The upper leg, which is the one to be tested, is placed in abduction, slight extension, and slight external rotation by the examiner, and the subject is asked to hold this position against pressure. Then the examiner uses one hand to help stabilize the pelvis while with the other he presses downward and slightly anteriorly on the lower part of the leg. Attempts by the subject to compensate by rotating the leg back into a neutral position, by rolling the upper hip backward or forward, or by bringing the thigh into flexion are common. The grade should be determined by the ability to hold against varying degrees of pressure in the designated test position. Tests for gluteus medius strength are of particular importance in cases of low back pain and in case of faulty alignment of the lower extremity.

Test of Gluteus Maximus
For this test the subject is in a prone position. With the knee bent to 90° or more the thigh is raised several inches above the table and the subject is asked to hold this position as downward pressure is exerted by the examiner on the lower part

of the posterior thigh.

Testing for strength of the gluteus maximus is of particular importance in cases of anterior pelvic tilt and in cases of coccyalgia.

With the subject prone, the knee is bent to about a 45° angle. The subject is asked to maintain the position of knee flexion as the examiner exerts downward pressure on the back of the ankle. **Test of Hamstring Muscles**

Test for strength of hamstrings is of special importance in cases of anterior pelvic tilt and hyperextension of the knees.

The subject is prone with the knee flexed to at least a 90° angle. The foot is placed in plantar flexion and the subject is asked to hold that position. The examiner provides support for the leg with one hand while with the other he exerts pressure to pull the heel towards the planta. **Test of Soleus**

This test is important for cases in which there is a deviation of the body forward from the plumb line. It is also advisable to test this muscle in cases in which there is an increase in the height of the longitudinal arch.

The test movement for the flexor hallucis longus is flexion of the distal joint of the big toe. The subject attempts to hold the position as the examiner applies pressure against the distal phalanx. **Tests for Toe Flexor Muscles**

For the flexor digitorum longus test the subject bends the distal joints of the second, third, fourth and fifth toes and holds against pressure by the examiner.

In pronation of the foot, weakness is frequently found in these two muscles. They are more often weaker on the left than on the right because the left foot is generally more pronated than the right.

The flexor brevis is tested by having the subject flex the toes and hold against pressure applied to the middle phalanx.

The test for flexor brevis is important in cases of longitudinal arch strain. A point of acute tenderness is often observed at the place of origin of this muscle on the os calcis.

In the test for flexion by the lumbricales the subject flexes the metatarsal-phalangeal joints of the four outer toes and holds while pressure is applied against the proximal phalanges.

Tests for strength of lumbricales are particularly important in cases of metatarsal arch strain and in cases of hammer toes.

A number of patterns of postural deviation can result from, or in, particular muscle weakness. Where the pelvis is tilted anteriorly, producing a lordotic lumbar spine and an elevated thoracic cage, the rectus abdominis lying between the pubic bone and the sternum will be stretched and weak.

In the postural condition where the pelvis is tilted anteriorly and the hips are held in flexion with a hyperextended or lordotic lumbar spine, with a compensating dorsal kyphosis, there will be tension, tightness and great strength in the low back extensors and hip flexors while the muscles controlling the lower abdomen and the hamstrings will be stretched and weak.

In the half-stooped posture in which the legs are deviated posteriorly and the trunk has deviated anteriorly with a compensatory anterior tilt of the pelvis, the hip joint is in flexion and the lumbar spine slightly hyperextended. The hip flexors will have shortened and the back extensors will be contracted. Where there exists a flattened lumbar curve due to a pelvic tilt posteriorly, there is often a tightness in the hamstrings and weakness in the hip flexors or back extensors or both. The abdominal muscles may or may not be strong and tight.

Where the pelvis and upper legs have swayed forward in relation to the feet there will be hyperextension of the hip. The pelvis will be tilted slightly posteriorly and there is no increase in the lumbar curve. The anterior hip ligaments, the hip flexor and the external oblique abdominal muscles limit and maintain this position. All these will be stretched and weak. The low back and hamstring muscle will be short and strong. The upper back muscles will be weak and stretched and the upper abdominals will be strong and short.

Where the pelvis deviates right and tilts to the left, the right hip is in adduction.

The right gluteus medius will be weaker than the left. The left leg is in abduction and the left hip adbuctors, especially the tensor fascia lata, will be tight and strong.

If the individual has marked weakness of the right gluteus medius muscle the trunk will deviate towards the affected leg causing an abduction of the right leg and excessive weight bearing on it.

The relevance of these conditions and any muscular weaknesses that might be ascertained should be correlated with tests to determine the physiological state of tightness of these same and others postural muscles. The length or tightness of these should be assessed by the following movements:

(a) The patient sitting and bending forward in an attempt to touch the fingers to the toes whilst keeping the knees straight. This tests the hamstrings, back extensors, gastrocnemius and soleus. A combination of changes in the muscles will produce a variety of results in this simple test.

(b) The straight leg raising tests is used to test the length of the hamstring muscles.

(c) The tensor fascia lata is assessed by the side-lying procedure in which the leg should be able to drop into adduction when the pelvis is fixed.

(d) The hip flexors are tested by one flexed leg being held in position whilst the thigh of the other leg, the lower part of which hangs over the table edge, is assessed to see whether the thigh remains in contact with the table. The iliopsoas, rectus femorus, tensor fascia lata and sartorius comprise this group. If the thigh maintains contact but the knee extends, preventing a free hanging lower leg then the rectus femorus is tight.

(e) The arms are stretched overhead to assess tightness of the adductor and internal rotator muscles. These include pectoralis major and minor, latissimus dorsi, teres major, subscapularis and the rhomboids. With the back flat and the knees flexed the arms should rest easily on the table above the head with the entire length of the arm in contact.

The testing of these muscles is not related to Goodheart's system Applied Kinesiology in which the weakness or otherwise of particular muscle groups is believed to indicate specific pathological states.

Objective assessment of the patient's posture combined with tests for muscle strength and muscle length (or tightness) provide the operator with the ability to concentrate on those areas of soft tissue dysfunction (too tight, too weak, too strong, too short etc.) which are present in any particular case. It should be borne in mind that posture represents not only the habitual manners of use, the occupational stresses and the inherited and acquired mechanical deviations but is also the mirror image of the total of psychic stress to which the individual has been and is being subjected. The degree of muscular guarding and built-in protective rigidity resulting from such stress presents a major area of dysfunction. The release of these tissues can often be of importance in normalizing emotional disturbances.

The operator has within the framework of the general and specific manoeuvres incorporated into NMT a method for dealing with the types of postural problems which result from or which cause soft tissue dysfunction. It goes without saying that other methods can and should be used as well in the ultimate correction of these conditions. These methods may include exercise, re-education, manipulation, corrective footwear etc. as indicated by the particular circumstances.

The use of NMT however gives an unequalled method for the normalizing and assessing of the soft tissue component.

A pattern of treatments over a series of ten to fifteen visits aimed at normalizing the spinal, abdominal and lower limb soft tissues, will effectively prepare the body for the correction of postural habits.

Rolfing techniques, which attempt to achieve similar results in eight treatment sessions, are notoriously painful, albeit successful. NMT need hurt no more than in a transient manner and it is at least as effective as Rolfing.

It is suggested that for postural correction, the first visit should deal with basic spinal and abdominal work, clearing up whatever is most obviously tense, contracted and painful. Following sessions should deal with the connective tissues and muscles of the feet and legs, the shoulders and the thorax, before returning to the spinal and abdominal tissues. Special emphasis should be applied to those soft tissues which postural patterns or muscle stretch or strength tests indicate to be most in need. After eight to ten sessions the patient should be demonstrably improved and retesting will give proof of this. At this stage postural re-education, exercises and breathing techniques all come into play. Until a moderate degree of soft tissue improvement has been achieved by this earlier treatment such additional measures would have less chance of success.

Stretching and Strengthening Exercises

The following exercises will prove useful in stretching or strengthening particular muscles and groups as indicated in any given case.

Exercises should be done daily until normal length has been restored to tight muscles and until weak muscles have been strengthened. There will always be both weakness and tightness in opposing groups of muscles and both aspects must be dealt with. NMT provides the ability to normalize those aspects of the soft tissues that cannot easily be improved by exercise alone, no matter how specific these may be.

Low Back Stretching Exercise Patient lies, face down, with a firm pillow under the abdomen and a small pillow or rolled towel under the ankles. The patient should relax in this position and then roll the pelvis inferiorly over the abdominal pillow by pulling down with the buttocks and hamstrings. The patient is trying to flatten the lumbar curve by tilting the pelvis posteriorly.

Lower Abdominal Exercise (1) Patient lies supine with a rolled towel under the knees. The hands are placed behind the neck and the patient tilts the pelvis posteriorly to flatten the low back against the surface. This is achieved by pulling the lower abdominal muscles up and in and holding this tension with the back flat whilst respiration continues deeply and slowly. The upper abdominal muscles should be relaxed and the chest should expand freely whilst the retracted muscles are held for at least a minute.

Lower Abdominal Exercise (2) The position is as above but with the knees bent and feet close to buttocks. The back is held flat as the legs are slowly slid into a straight position. The back should remain flat during this manoeuvre and also as the knees resume the bent position, one at a time. Repeat eight to ten times.

Upper Abdominal Exercise Patient lies on the back with a rolled towel under the knees and the pelvis tilted to flatten the lower spine. The arms are extended forward or placed behind the head and the patient lifts the head and shoulders approximately ten inches (25cm) from the surface and slowly returns to a lying position. Repeat eight to ten times.

Pectoral Stretch Exercise Patient lies on the back, knees bent and the low back held flat to the surface, one or both arms are stretched above the head. The entire length of the arm should touch the surface with the elbow straight and as close to the side of the head as possible. This position is held for at least a minute while the patient breaths and relaxes.

Low Back and Hamstring Stretch Patient sits with legs extended and a rolled towel under the knees. The abdominal muscles are retracted and the patient reaches forward to grasp the toes (or the furthest point of the legs possible). This should cause a degree of stretch in the low back area and the back of the legs. This should be repeated ten to fifteen times and then maintained for at least a minute to complete the exercise.

Hamstring Stretch Same position as above but without towel under the knees.

Anterolateral Thigh Stretch The patient adopts a position similar to that of an athlete at the start of a sprint. The foot of the flexed leg should be placed on the floor and remain flat whilst the foot of the leg which extends posteriorly should be dorsiflexed and internally rotated so that weight is born on the ball of the foot. The hands are placed on the floor immediately below the head. The major tension is applied to the antero-lateral aspect of the thigh by flexing the forward knee so that the pelvis is moved down. A rocking motion is maintained to repetitively stretch these structures. It is important for the knee on the extended leg to remain fully extended during the exercise which should be repeated slowly and strongly fifteen to twenty times.

Upper Back Trapezius Stretch (1)

The patient sits on a stool with the back against a wall. The hands should be placed palm forward beside the head. The low back should be flattened against the wall by retracting the abdominal muscles. An effort to push the body against the wall is made whilst of the head is stretched upwards with the chin pressed in and back. The elbows should be pressed back against the wall. This position should be maintained for not less than one minute.

Upper Back and Trapezius Stretch (2)

The same position as above should be adopted but this time with the arms upwards and outwards so that they are stretched diagonally away from the midline at about 45° from the vertical. This position (abdomen retracted, chin in and crown of the head up) should be maintained for at least a minute. A few variations in arm position, to bring them directly above the head and then return to the diagonal position should be carried out during the exercise.

Muscle Balance and Lumbosacral Flexion Exercise

The patient stands with feet twelve inches (30cm) apart and with the feet externally rotated to an angle of about 30° from the parallel. The heels remain flat on the floor throughout. In women accustomed to high heels this will not be possible and in this event shoes should be worn. At no point during this exercise should the patient rise onto the toes. The spine should be flexed with head bowed, the arms should be pointed to the floor at a point between the toes.

A 'flat-footed' squat is then performed so that the buttocks approximate the heels and the fingers touch the floor, elbows between the knees. If there is a tendency to overbalance (as will be the case with long-femured individuals) a counter balance of about 8 lbs (3½ kg) may be held. By attempting to reach the desired position repeatedly (ten to fifteen times) a degree of stretching will occur in the lumbosacral area and in the posterior calf. The quadriceps femoris and gluteus maximus will be strengthened.

Having reached the position of squatting, an up and down jigging movement is useful—this can be thought of as trying to 'tuck the tail between the legs'.

Foot and Knee Stretch

The patient stands with feet straight forward about two inches (5cm) apart. The knees should be relaxed, neither rigid nor bent. The foot and calf muscles that raise the arch should be contracted and the weight should be transferred slightly to the outer borders of the feet. The buttocks should be tightened to externally rotate the legs to the degree that allows the knees to point directly forward. This is to be repeated ten to fifteen times.

Depending upon the indications the appropriate exercises should be performed daily.

Conclusion In the long run posture can only be corrected by the individual learning afresh how to use his body machines correctly. The breaking of old habits and the learning of new ones is not easy but the employment of NMT to normalize the soft tissues will increase the individuals awareness of his body's structures whilst at the same time removing restrictions which can often physically prevent correct use of a part of the body. If one part malfunctions then the whole will malfunction. In earlier chapters we have seen how posture, tension, dysfunction and emotional states are often intertwined. By breaking into this web of interconnecting factors and releasing soft tissue structures from the contractions and patterns of stress imposed upon them, many of the other aspects of the problem will become.more easily soluble. Thus with soft tissue relaxation comes the chance for postural improvement as well as a re-education in muscular tension patterns and a reduction of fatigue and those psychological tension states that feed on these physical conditions.

In treating an individual for postural dysfunction the basic spinal and abdominal treatments are used as well as all the other techniques (tissue release, elbow technique, skin rolling etc.), as and when the indications are found. Not only should tight groups and areas be stretched and normalized but the weak, overstretched areas should be exercised and toned as part of the process of normalization.

[1]Page, Dr Leon, *Academy of Applied Osteopathy Yearbook* (1952).
[2]Jones, Lawrence, *The Postural Complex,* (Charles Thomas, Springfield, Illinois, 1955).
[3]Kendall, Kendall and Boynton, *Posture and Pain,* (The Williams and Wilkins Co., Baltimore, 1952).

Chapter 8

On Energy

A variety of systems and methods have concepts of energy which differ from the normally accepted concept of this phenomenon. Energy lost or wasted by the maintenance of unnecessary muscular and fascial tension is easily demonstrable. That such a situation is undesirable is also clear for, if maintained, such a drain on energy can lead to local and general fatigue of pathological significance, as well as creating a 'feedback' by which psychic tensions are reinforced. This self-maintenance of tension states makes the recognition of the somatico-psychic aspect of pathology causation as important as that which attaches to the psycho-somatic component.

Energy interference has been theorized by a number of individuals and systems. Some of these will be briefly considered since, if their theories are valid, in whole or part, then the significance to a method such as NMT is obvious. In releasing neuro-muscular contraction and tensions much more may be taking place than is realized.

Varma,[1] who gave Stanley Lief the original idea for NMT stated his views, which were derived from traditional Ayurvedic philosophy, as follows:

Vibration is the manifestation and movement of life—it is life itself. The source of all vibration is the universal force known as the *prana,* of which the most tangible manifestations are the ultra-sensitive currents of the atmosphere.

The average number of vibrations for man is 360 per second, the proportion being much higher in the head than in the feet. Thus, varying degrees of high frequency and low frequency can be recorded throughout the body from the top of the head to the tips of the fingers and the toes.

These currents provide the body with varying degrees of heat in order to regulate the density of its fluid content.

We have discovered that our bodies pick up two kinds of currents at two points: the ultra-sensitive currents at the pineal gland; and the sensitive currents at the nerve fibres below the cranium.

The ultra-sensitive vibrations, starting from the pineal gland in the middle of the encephalus, pursue a circular route, passing through back and front (spinal cord and sternum), to the middle of the body. This produces a kind of circuit with two poles, the pineal gland and the cocygeal plexus. Between these two poles, the currents flow downwards to stimulate the different organs, and upwards to inform the brain of heat or cold, pain or oversenitivity. The stoppage of circulation in any part, irritation or other pathological phenomena such as indigestion, stiffness of joints and all the ailments of a disordered nervous system—every form of abnormal condition is communicated to the brain by the returning flow of sensitive currents.

If adhesions of muscular fibres occur in the region of the atlas, this current cannot pass easily, and the body suffers from the deficiency. In cases of very obstructive adhesions it is cut off, just as in the case of a 'blown' electric fuse, and the body dies.

On either side of the spinal column, from the atlas to the coccyx, we find sympathetic nerve-ganglia, which are protected by muscular fibres. These ganglia act as electric batteries which are charged with the descending current and which distribute this current to the right and left to the various organs.

Special mention may well be made of the sensitivity current which is to be found in the first of the four layers of the skin. If the latter is in normal condition, the nervous current passes freely through the nerve fibres, but if the skin becomes attached to the underlying muscle, the current cannot pass, the part loses its sensibility and is said to be paralysed.

It may be stated as a general rule that all illnesses are caused through some kind of disorder in the flow of nervous current. Such disorders are generally caused by adhesions of the muscular fibres. These adhesions may arise suddenly through an accident (such as crushing by a heavy object) or gradually, through constant exercise of a single part of the body, or through exposure to draughts or damp, causing the skin to adhere to the muscles. Such adhesions, though slight at first, obstruct the passage of the nervous current; the adhesion consequently becomes more obstinate, until, finally the passage of the nervous current becomes completely blocked, the tissues fail to be reproduced, and the organ in question loses its suppleness.

Albert Abrams M.D. the father of the 'Black Box', and either a genius or a lunatic, depending upon the entrenched viewpoint from which his ideas are examined, states his views as follows: [2]

Everything in nature is in a state of perpetual motion and the latter is continually changing from one velocity to another.

The power to change the state of motion of a body is *energy*. The total energy contained in matter depends on the extent to which it can be changed. Energy is the universal commodity on which all life depends.

All forms of energy, whether derived from heat, electricity, magnetism or gravitation are interconvertible and represent practically different varieties of motion. Energy, like matter, can neither be created nor destroyed. The first principle of energetics is, all physical phenomena (vital or chemical), are forms of motion. All these forms are susceptible to or change into one another, and in all the transformations the quantity of mechanical work represented by different modes of motions remains invariable. Atomic energy, like matter, in accordance with the Law of the Conservation of Energy, is indestructible and uncreatable. Energy is differentiated as *potential and kinetic.*

Our present conception of matter presumes a cyclic or vibratory motion of electrons and it continues as potential energy until transformed into actual energy by some exciting energy from without.

Every living being is a transformer of energy converting the environmental energy into mechanical motion, heat and nervous energy.

Investigations of all ages have espoused the theory of *human radiations.*

To some the organism is compared to a Voltaic battery which emits something akin to electricity.

The hagiologist conciliates the reality of radiations by referring to the auras in ancient pictures around the heads and bodies of Christ and the saints. The phenomena of light in materialization have been witnessed and accepted by notable scientists as spiritual phenomena. Of superstition, it has been said, that it is true psychology with the wrong dress.

The writer is convinced that the phenomena are realities independent of disembodied spirits and can be referred to the manifestations of human energy. Disocculting the occult will be possible when one attains a better understanding of the activities of living cells and when the biologist knows the laws that govern cell growth with the accuracy of the scientist knowing his laws. Every individual, it is maintained, is enveloped in a radiance (aura) invisible to the carnal eye and only perceived by the soul accustomed to it. Perception of the aura is the supposed prerogative of clairvoyance but Kilner has shown that any one can observe the 'atmosphere' surrounding the human body by aids of chemical screens, notably one containing a solution of dicyanin which, by partially paralyzing the retinal rods and cones causes visibility of the aura in a darkened room.

Philosophism, the refuge of the scientifically destitute, can never substitute objectivity in scientific research.

There are more false facts than theories and the true scientist does not hesitate to preside at a birth of a theory and officiate at its burial on the morrow. Energy liberated by the organism appears in mechanical, thermal and electrical form.

The human generates electricity statically by muscular movement.

The body may be likened to a collection of storage cells, which are liable to become highly charged, or to have their charge altered by any direct or passing current, or exciting influence. Electromotive force continues even when the body is absolutely motionless, hence the theory of chemical generation of nerve force. Electricity in the body must be constantly discharged, otherwise the electrical pressure would become unbearable. The skin, the body insulator, is not of uniformly high resistance. Sign, electromotive force and current vary with the individual. Whereas the generation of electricity in the body may be constant, its dissipation cannot be so by reason of the varying conditions of external conductivity.

Abrams went into the field of radionic diagnosis and treatment and his contribution to physical therapy included the recognition of reflex areas for diagnostic purposes and spondylotherapy, the percussion of the spinal centres, to create a vibratory response on the part of the body. The author cannot resist the temptation to quote one more paragraph from Abrams book:

Why does the physician fail to recognize disease in its incipiency? Owing to the arbitary domination of the cell theory, he awaits cellular alterations which are *effects*. Disease in its incipiency is only a physiological disturbance. Just as the barometer portends a storm so may these cellular alterations be anticipated and checked. The phenomena of disease are not inert but dynamic. Thus the actions of the body should be regarded as processes and not as structures and, if the microscope is utilized as a criterion of disease when cell changes have ensued, the patient is eligible for the morgue and not the hospital.

Not, it would seem, the words of a lunatic! The concept of an energy discharge from areas of lowered skin resistance and of an 'aura' surrounding the body finds its echoes in modern electro-acupuncture and Kirlian photography.

Polarity   Dr Randolph Stone has elaborated upon these ideas and has evolved a system of
Therapy   soft tissue and bony manipulation which is designed to restore energy balance.
He has called this Polarity Therapy. He states: [3]

> In this atomic age of science we realize that matter itself is but a mass of spinning
> energy particles which appear as solid substances. In reality, they exist as such only
> because of a constant flow of energy currents between all parts and portions. As soon
> as that circuit is interrupted, changes begin to appear which, in the human body, are
> interpreted as pain or disease. The interrupted current cannot reach the core to flow
> through and out again. In the meantime, the opposing currents pile up energy
> particles at the point of interruption and act as blocks in the area where they occur.
> This pressure of energy particles in any of the five fields of matter registers as intense
> pain, or obstruction of normal energy flow, called disease.

To give an idea of his therapeutic methods the following is illustrative: [4]

> Correlate the function of the vital centres through the re-establishment of polarity in
> the parasympathetic and sympathetic nervous systems by *Perineal and Polarity*
> contacts and techniques.
>   Rule. No relaxation of the voluntary nervous system and muscles can occur as long
> as the involuntary muscles are locked and tense. *No bony correction should be forced.*
> Merely telling the patient to relax, is useless.
>   Have the patient lie on the left side on a soft table, with the head on a pillow, knees
> drawn up. The operator sits on a stool, facing the back of the patient. Trace the path
> of vital forces in their *bipolar* action, from the neck to the perineum.
>   Check the neck for tenderness and spastic muscles; with the left hand contact the
> sorest spot, and either inhibit or stimulate firmly (whichever happens to be indicated)
> over the lamina.
>   With the first or second finger of the right hand, find the most tender spot in the
> perineum, on the same side of the neck lesion. Use a finger cot on the finger of this
> hand, or work through thin clothing, such as a gown or underwear. Take care *never to
> enter an orifice when giving this treatment,* because the nerve endings we are
> balancing now are on the surface.
>   If the pulse is fast, the upper cervical area—or any sore spot over the occipital
> space—is lightly and slowly stimulated by a double contact, rotary movement; this
> applies to neck contact in general. Because this is a vagus area, you are balancing the
> pulse with the two nervous systems. Most pulses are fast because of habitual tension
> and over-strenuous, hurried living. In these cases, the ropy neck muscles can be slowly
> manipulated while the Perineal Contact is held.
>   If the pulse is slow, inhibit the tender neck areas, and further check the carotid pulse
> of each side of normalization each time after the two contacts are held, until the pulse
> is improved.
>   If the pulse is normal, the rule for general treatment applies:
>   First, inhibit the most tender area gently, then more firmly. This is the principle of
> 'Yin' inhibition, or drawing off energy.
>   Second, use heavy pressure or stimulation on the less tender area or constricted
> area; namely, the principle of 'Yang', to tonify.
>   Make firm contact with the most tender perineal spot found. The neck and the
> perineum are contacted *simultaneously.* Regardless of pulse, the perineal contact is
> made with *one finger,* and is an *upward lift* (toward the head or neck contact, on the
> same side). This lift is increased as relaxation allows it. If the perineum is flaccid and
> relaxed, then it needs tone and stimulative contacts, by repeated *upward* impacts on
> the contact.

Any sharp, pin-sticking sensation here, like a finger nail or knife point is due to crystallized deposits or other products of chemistry, which were carried along by the energy currents in the short-circuiting effect. It is the action of a local cataphoresis. A few inhibitions will cause this to be re-absorbed by the circulation, and carried away, as the short-circuiting is stopped and energy flows in regular paths again. When nerve relaxation occurs the spinal muscles also relax, and previous occipital and dorsal findings will have changed.

The work of Stone incorporates both the Chinese Yin/Yang concept and the Hindu *prana* concept.

Yin and Yang

In Taoist thinking all phenomena are activated by the movement of energy, the opposite poles of which are known as Yin and Yang. The interaction between these two forces is seen in human terms in, for example, the spirallic formation of the embryo and the relationship between various structures and functions. Yin and Yang are seen to operate via the medium of dynamic energy called *chi*. Harmonious flow of this energy is thought to be the prime requirement for health. In such a state the organism vibrates in harmony with its environment. The restoration of this balance is the aim of Oriental medicine in general and acupuncture in particular. Yin and Yang may be thought of as low frequency and high frequency waves respectively. There is said to be a fluctuation of the energy potential in the various body 'meridians' at different times of the day. Thus, each meridian or channel of energy has a period of maximum potential and therefore a period at which time treatment would be more likely to be of benefit. This may sound far fetched but the reader should consider the recent American findings that medication has an optimum time for its effective consumption by the individual. Different body systems have their optimum periods of activity. The study of this phenomenon by orthodox science is called chrono-biology.

Acupuncture points may be located by the measurement of the electrical potential of the skin surface. They will be found in areas of low resistance, and these areas will also be demonstrated (in Kirlian photography for example) as areas of high energy discharge. In active pathological conditions or when dysfunction has occurred these areas will also be sensitive to pressure. The relevance of soft tissue techniques becomes apparent when we realize that pressure on acupuncture points is often just as effective as needling or electrical stimulation. It is also relevant to our study to realize that all these acupuncture points lie within the muscles and fascia and many of them are identical with reflexes discovered by others and which are amenable to techniques used in NMT treatment.

The Aura

Kirlian photography is a technique using high-voltage photography. The developed plates show a luminescence or pattern of electrical discharge emanating from the entire body surface. Various interpretations have been made as to the significance of this electrical 'aura'. From the viewpoint of this study the importance is that it verifies as fact the existence of some sort of electro-magnetic discharge on the part of the body which is influenced by the state of health of the individual and by therapy, of whatever sort.

The influence may not always be to the benefit of the body and the patterns of discharge will vary accordingly. The verification of acupuncture points as areas of greater discharge is also significant, especially as these areas can be shown to become more or less active in different pathological states, and further that they can be seen to be more or less sensitive to pressure at the same times. In attempting to reach an understanding of the acupuncture phenomenon I have quoted from the work of Speransky, in my book *The Acupuncture Treatment of Pain*.[5]

In his study of the nature of disease, Speransky explained how, after years of research, he became convinced that, in studying the processes of disease, the traditional subdivision of the nervous system into central, peripheral, sympathetic etc. had no justification. He showed in many experiments that, from any point in the nervous system, it was possible to bring into action nerve mechanisms, the functioning of which terminated at the periphery, producing changes of a bio-physico-chemical character.

He developed the thesis that any nerve point, not excluding peripheral nerve structures, could become the originator of neuro-dystrophic processes serving as the temporary or permanent nerve centre of these processes, and pointed out that whenever a procedure affected the nervous aspect of any phenomenon, the resultant changes were not only in the nerve portion concerned, but in the whole intricate complex. Also apparent from his work was the fact that irritation of any points of the nervous system could evoke changes, not only in the adjacent parts, but also in remote regions of the organism.

Finally, he stated that it became evident that the usefulness of operating on the nervous system was often due to the very act of interference itself and not to its form, whilst harm depended on its form and was associated with excessive trauma. I find in these thoughts of Speransky's the justification for my views on acupuncture and, in a large part, the explanation for the acupuncture phenomenon.

Rolfing A system of physical therapy that incorporates a concept of energy being 'locked' in the body in states of disease and being released by therapy is that developed by Ida Rolf. 'Rolfing' recognizes a total mind/body interaction and sees this reflected in the musculoskeletal component of the body where a degree of shielding or armouring takes place to protect the individual from emotional discomforts, as well as from the conscious experience of inner hurts, that accumulate throughout life. A further concept of Rolfing is that gravity not only upholds man but that it 'feeds' him. It sees therapy as designed to release energies locked up in the armour or defence mechanism and to balance (posturally) the individual so that the forces of gravity can act and support him.

The importance of energy locked into the musculoskeletal tissues was demonstrated by Eeman.[6] His work, which was similar in direction to that of Abrams and Stone, clearly showed that without neuro-muscular relaxation there could not be mento-emotional relaxation. This observation can now be demonstrated by measuring brain wave patterns in varying stages of physical relaxation.

Cooper[7] echoes Rolf's ideas and adds some additional thoughts of some significance. He points out that osteopathic practitioners have observed and recorded the extent to which all degenerative changes in the body are reflected in the superficial fascia. Any degree of degeneration changes the nature of fascia. As this elastic envelope is stretched, manipulative mechanical energy is added to it and fascial colloid softens to become more gel-like and less solid. He states:

It is an accepted fact that life happens only where there is protoplasm behaving colloidally. In living structures the colloids are extremely sensitive, with enormous possibilities with regard to stability and reversibility of phase. One of the characteristics of life is periodicity or rhythmicity, in other words, fluctuation between predominance of sol and gel phases.

In an organism living in health, the complex totality of manifold colloidal structures behaves with appropriate periodicity and rhythm between certain phase limits. Any phase of any of the colloidal systems which goes beyond the appropriate limit or fails to reach the limit within the proper time will affect the health of the organism as a whole. Likewise any factor, intrinsic or extrinsic, capable of altering colloidal behaviour will have a marked effect one way or another on the welfare of the organism. Physical colloidal states so paired with nervous, mental, and other characteristics and illnesses are connected with colloidal disturbances.

He goes on to point out that colloids may be influenced by five factors, i.e. physical (e.g. heat), biological (e.g. bacteria), chemical (e.g. drugs). psychic (e.g. practitioner's intention; emotion) and mechanical (e.g. pressure or friction).

Taylor[8] points out that:

It is the law of the physical universe that every system, if left to itself, changes spontaneously either slowly or rapidly in such a way as to approach a definite final state of rest or equilibrium. Likewise, it is also a law of the universe that, once this state of rest or equilibrium has been reached, no reverse change or moving away from equilibrium can be brought about without the application of some form of energy. This is the thermodynamic concept and is simply stated: a system and its surroundings are in equilibrium in such a way that any change in the energy of the system will result in a change in the energy of its surroundings.

Lawson-Wood has written widely on energy in relation to health and he states in regard to colloidal states:[9]

All life is found in the colloidal form; and there are many forms of 'gel' which have been in that state of 'gel' for a very long time and are unlikely to do other than continue the slow ageing process but which are nevertheless reversible if energy of the right kind can be applied.

Cooper and Lawson-Wood insist on the importance of operators visualizing his intention and the desired end-result of their manipulative or soft tissue treatment. This they maintain will have an effect on the colloidal state. Becker[10] makes the important additional comment on the value of the patient's consciousness being incorporated into the therapy programme in whatever dysfunction there might be. He gives the following example:

To illustrate the matter of changing the programme an individual has installed to resist a postural imbalance due to anatomical inequality in the lower extremeties: Since the programme was established to maintain body balance on an uneven base, it is obvious that simply placing a lift under the short leg will increase the problem because the programme is automatic. The muscle pulls that served to maintain balance on an uneven base will be inappropriate under the new circumstances and will create further imbalance unless the individual is trained to reprogramme the computer (i.e. his mind). So the physician explains to the patient how the new balance will affect her actions, uses whatever methods he prefers to equalize muscle tensions and fascial pulls and correct or release any impairments in articular motion, teaches the patient to cancel the old programmes by consciously releasing the muscles each time before she starts a new action and gives her some controlled exercises which call into play new standards or proprioceptive data which now will define the normal, acceptable and tolerable limits.

Becker goes on to comment on residual patterns of soft tissue stress following a traumatic incident, namely, a whiplash injury.

Here the problem is complicated by the fact that the body has been subjected to forces that entered it in a direction that crosses the normal direction of movement. Such forces tend to produce a wave-like movement within the fluid cells of the body, and the inertia of the body, which is trying to continue whatever programmes are in action at the time, causes a counterwave directed toward the point of impact. The resultant of these two sets of force vectors produces a standing wave, or ridge of energy, a kind of built-in distortion, around which the defensive programmes are installed. If the physician attempts to remove this distortion, the body activates the protective mechanisms or programmes unless the physician first dissipates this ridge of energy by appropriate manipulative means. In other words, the energy of impact and the counter-energy of resistance must be permitted to pass through each other rather than opposing one another, and then the programmes in the CNS computer which were designed to operate around this built-in distortion must be cancelled and new ones established to include the new energy.

Energy means different things to different people. Simple stress patterns locked into the soft tissues as a result of trauma or postural or emotional factors will reduce the energy potentials of the individual. Release will encourage normalization and will reduce the drain on vital energy. That is the simplistic view and if that is all that is involved it is of great value.

If, however, there do exist more subtle energy transactions which soft tissue dysfunction can interrupt then the value of the restoration of balance in this regard will be of immense value. The reader must solve the riddle to his own satisfaction. The quest for greater knowledge in this field will lead to many strange abstruse byways of human research and endeavour. That something akin to an energy field surrounds the body is not really the question. What is to be clearly established is that the existence of this has relevance to the field of health in general and manipulative therapy in particular.

[1] Varma, Dewanchand, *The Human Machine and Its Forces,* (Health For All Publishing Co., 1930).

[2] Abrams, Dr Albert, *New Concepts in Diagnosis and Treatment,* (Physico-clinical Co., San Francisco, 1922).

[3] Stone, Randolph, *Polarity Therapy,* (privately published, 1954).

[4] Stone, Randolph, *The New Energy Concept,* (privately published, 1948).

[5] Chaitow, Leon, *The Acupuncture Treatment of Pain,* (Thorsons, 1976).

[6] Eeman, L., *Co-operative Healing,* (Frederick Muller, 1947).

[7] Cooper, Gerald J., *Journal of the American Osteopathic Association,* Vol. 78, pp. 336-73 (January, 1979).

[8] Taylor, R. B., 'Bio-energetics of Man', *Academy of Applied Osteopathy Yearbook,* 1958, p. 91.

[9] Lawson-Wood, D. and J., *Progressive Vitality and Dynamic Posture,* (Health Science Press, 1978).

[10] Becker, Alan R., 'Parameters of Resistance', *Journal of the American Osteopathic Association* (September, 1973), p. 39.

Chapter 9

NMT in Clinical Use

The holistic, total, approach to the problems of man's health is one which looks to the causes of dysfunction and disease and, by removing these, allows the homeostatic efforts of the body to restore normality. This ideal is not always attainable but remains the aim. Each individual has an optimum degree of biomechanical (structural, postural, functional), biochemical and psychological efficiency that can be realized. It is this optimum that is being aimed for in all therapies that fall into the broad net of holistic healing methods.

NMT takes its place amongst these methods since its objective is to help to restore the structural, functional and postural integrity of the body by removing restrictions and aiding in the normalization of dysfunction. NMT aids the economy and functional ability of the body further by reducing self-perpetuating stress factors such as contractions, spasms and tensions in the soft tissue components of the system. By improving function, removing pain, reducing energy loss, improving posture etc. the effect on psychologically negative states is a positive one.

In itself NMT is only a tool, a useful method or technique which can be of immense use in a variety of conditions. It possesses one further criterion which places it firmly in the holistic armamentary. This being that it does nothing to the body which is harmful to its overall state of health i.e. it has no side-effects. Indeed by normalizing the soft tissues NMT often saves the individual from techniques of a more 'violent' nature which might well produce outward reactions, such as surgery, traction, immobilization etc., and techniques which, whilst not usually harmful, can be painful, such as manipulative joint techniques.

NMT has an immense capability for diagnostic application, and since this can take place at the same time as its therapeutic application it shows economy in the use of time and energy. Since NMT is entirely a manual technique it is not wasteful of resources such as heat, power etc. and is applicable under almost any circumstances or conditions. NMT may be universally applied to any patient of any age suffering from any condition. This is not to say that it will be curative or even of marked value in all conditions. But it will be of some diagnostic and some therapeutic value in every condition and of enormous value in others, since no one is free of some degree of dysfunction, which affects the overall efficiency and economy of the body.

In general terms, NMT may be applied to all cases of musculoskeletal dysfunction and mento-emotional dysfunction with benefit. The basic spinal and basic abdominal techniques are used as diagnostic and therapeutic tools in the majority of cases. The more specific techniques such as psoas, piriformis and abdominal release techniques are used as and when indicated. A general, full body NMT treatment may be applied as part of a programme of postural re-integration.

In specific terms NMT is applied as follows. All conditions of the spine and conditions which involve the arms or legs would receive general spinal technique as well as consideration of local areas, in the limbs affected. Such treatments would be repeated once or twice weekly until a degree of normality had been achieved. As should be obvious, other modalities and techniques would and should be used if called for. NMT combines with anything of a supportive nature which is aimed at the restoration of normal function, such as (in appropriate conditions) ultrasonic therapy, diathermy, manipulation etc.

At the outset the aim of general treatment is to remove the more obvious areas of contraction and stasis. All reflex trigger points should be neutralized by pressure techniques if possible or, if found stubborn, by vapo-coolant or even infiltration methods. As therapy progresses, individual patterns of dysfunction will become clear and more specific NMT would be applied to those spinal, abdominal, intercostal and pelvic areas slow to improve.

Manipulative techniques of a non-specific type are often useful in the normalization of spinal integrity once the initial soft tissue rigidity or dysfunction has been improved. NMT may be applied with infinite gentleness or with robust enthusiasm since it is possible to use the same techniques with a marked difference in the degree of force employed. This enables its application to areas of acute sensitivity as well as in fragile (osteoporotic) and tender areas. As long as the operator is thinking about the task in hand and not applying the techniques in a mechanical, repetitive manner there is no danger of injury or harm.

If treatment is aimed at the removal of symptoms stemming from trigger points, it is essential to normalize all the structures related to the local area of dysfunction. To simply neutralize the trigger that is causing, say, a headache, will produce short-term benefits. If the particular trigger lies in the trapezius muscle then not only must the trigger be normalized and the trapezius treated but the entire cervical and spinal musculature and soft tissues must receive attention. A general rule should be that *no part of the whole should be considered without the whole also being considered.* Thus, even if the spinal areas are receiving the main attention of the therapist on any one visit, the supporting limbs and associated structures should be given some, if only brief, consideration to assess their involvement and possible requirements. The treatment of the back, therefore, calls for the treatment of the front and this calls for the whole to be considered and treated.

General abdominal technique is useful in all cases of digestive and intestinal dysfunction of a non-organic nature. NMT is applicable to all cases of respiratory dysfunction. It is also applicable to all genito-urinary conditions of a non-organic nature. NMT applied to the abdomen will reduce dramatically most tension states of mento-emotional origin. General abdominal technique improves circulatory efficiency through the pelvis and abdominal regions and it improves respiratory function. The reflex points and zones in the spinal area should always be treated prior to thoracic and abdominal technique as indicated.

In a case of spastic constipation, for example, NMT to the lower spinal areas *(see Figure 2a)* and the use of neuro-lymphatic points *(see Figures 12a to 12e)* followed by general abdominal technique would be the pattern recommended. This could be followed by specific abdominal release techniques if areas of marked contractions or 'adhesion' were elicited during the general treatment. Such an approach, combined with general health measures, such as nutritional reform and an exercise and possibly a relaxation programme, will promote a return to normal more speedily than anything else in the author's experience. After all, the body is being given those factors required for normality and since its self-healing tendency is constantly acting, the removal of obstacles (structural, mechanical, dietary) provide the prerequisites for recovery.

In dealing with tension and stress of psychic origin it is as well to recall that the mind will not be calm or relaxed as long as neuro-muscular tensions are present. In applying any form of psychotherapy the use of NMT, applied to the spine and abdomen, will increasely improve the patient's powers of relaxation. NMT is not seen as an end in itself in this regard, but to be rather as a catalyst to the removal, albeit temporary, of the physical component of a vicious circle. In some cases this physical release of tension, especially when applied to the solar plexus, can produce a sudden emotional release in which the patient may cry and sob. The body becomes a solid mass of tensions and contractions for many individuals. The tensions of life are mirrored by layers of muscular 'armour'. The posture and tensions thus created all carry specific emotional charges and memories and as the physical components are broken down and relaxed so do the emotional memories and feelings associated with their origins come to the surface. NMT applied skillfully to the spine and abdomen becomes a useful tool for the therapist who is attempting to calm the mind of the patient. Tensions thus released do not return unless the causes are still current.

In restoring total structural and postural integrity to the body it is, of course, necessary to apply NMT to all the supporting structures of the body. This would involve the spinal, thoracic and abdominal soft tissues and the limbs, including the feet. NMT and manipulation, where appropriate, will lay the foundations for a return to normal (or to the patient's individual optimum norm). Specific and general exercise, as well as postural re-education, may then follow. It is possible, via such systems as Alexander Technique, to achieve postural and functional normality. It is contended, however, that by the judicious use of NMT and manipulation such re-education becomes much easier and less arduous. It must be easier to learn to use a machine correctly if that machine is capable of functioning correctly!

In attempting to achieve postural and functional normality a fairly long-term view is required. Some workers assert that a series of eight to ten sessions will produce this result. It is the author's experience that whilst the basic ground work can be done in eight to ten treatments, the majority of cases require weekly or fortnightly treatment for 12 to 18 months if they are to achieve optimum improvement. This should be followed by maintenance visits at not less than three monthly intervals.

NMT is universally applicable. It has no side-effects. It combines with all other methods of positive health care. In itself it is capable of improving general function, releasing tension and removing noxious triggers, which may be responsible for myriad symptoms. NMT has limits, but within the framework of its own area of application its only limits lie in the ability of the operator.

One practitioner who has achieved outstanding success in applying NMT to athletic injuries of marked severity is Terry G. Moule D.O. Within the last few years he has restored the former captain of England's soccer team, Gerry Francis, to playing fitness. Surgery to the lumbar spine was the only prospect left for Francis after months of agony under orthopaedic investigation. In desperation Moule was consulted and within a few weeks Francis was playing again. He remains fit and continues to play professional soccer.

A similar return to normality was achieved in the case of the then captain of England's rugby football team, Roger Uttley, whose career appeared to be over after a back injury. Treatment consisting largely of NMT has resulted in Uttley returning to the England squad in their successful 1980 season.

An even more startling result of the application of NMT to a spinal injury is that involving the current holder of the world mile and 1500m records Sebastian Coe. He stated in late 1979: 'Last winter I had a back problem. I was having trouble getting a diagnosis, let alone treatment.' Within a few treatments incorporating NMT he was running again and setting world record times. Moule has stated that he is not yet fully satisfied that Coe's back has reached its optimum improvement and he expects greater things still from this fine athlete.

Terry Moule's view of NMT is as follows:

The principle of NMT is that it is of prime importance to treat connective tissue lesions and abnormalities, prior to any manipulative treatment of the bony structures. If more orthodox and less penetrating soft tissue techniques are used, whilst the bony abnormality may be corrected by the application of a specific adjustment, because the soft tissues remain in a similar state to that existing prior to the manipulation, there is a strong likelihood of a recurrence of the lesion. NMT tends to dispense with specific adjustment, for, subsequent to using these specialized soft tissue measures, a generalized mobilization adjustment will allow the muscular and connective tissues to encourage the bony structures to return to their normal alignment. This may take a little longer to produce relief from discomfort, but in the long run it means that the correction is more permanent and there is less danger of any damage to the muscular and connective tissues from forceful manipulation.

The great advantage of NMT is that it may be applied to any part of the body. It is particularly effective in dealing with problems related to interference with nerve supply; to any form of muscular or connective tissue lesion; to treatment of the abdominal and pelvic organs etc. It is applied mainly by use of the thumb. It may take some years to develop an adequate 'feel' in the hands in general and the thumbs in particular, to effectively diagnose and treat lesions. It is the ability to diagnose through the thumb which is so helpful in the rapid and efficient treatment of all forms of dysfunction. Correctly used it precludes a large number of more conventional techniques and saves a considerable amount of time.

NMT has proved invaluable in the treatment of sports injuries, particularly for the diagnostic reasons outlined above and for the fact that it produces a rapid response as compared to orthodox soft tissue and physiotherapy techniques. With sports injuries one of the major problems is to get the player back in action as soon as possible, particularly where the injury is to a professional sportsman. NMT has been used very effectively on a large number of sportsmen and women following all types of sports.

One of the most common injuries one encounters is hamstring problems. These are particularly prevalent amongst footballers, who in many cases develop the injury through overdevelopment of the quadriceps without adequate attention to the maintenance and mobility (i.e. lengthening and stretching) of the hamstrings at the same time. The normal treatment of hamstring injuries is ultra-sonic and massage. These techniques are not particularly rapid and the resultant loss of overall muscle tone, due to the inability of the leg to be used normally, retards a return to normal function. With NMT a lesion can be accurately and rapidly detected and, by the use of deep thumb manipulation, the soft tissue lesion can be dealt with rapidly and effectively. Where there is muscular fibre damage this can be felt and literally ironed out. The effect of the technique is to stimulate circulation in the area thus encouraging healing. Where there is inflammation and swelling the technique promotes drainage and the restoration of normal tone. With acute lesions the technique is unfortunately painful, but where speed is the prime order in recovery this is a small price to pay.

NMT is also beneficial in the treatment of knee lesions, particularly ligamentous problems and the subsequent inflammation in the joint itself. Correct application of NMT to these lesions will improve drainage from the knee and encourages healing to take place far more rapidly than through orthodox techniques. Where there is knee misalignments or dislocation, reduction of spasm is most important as a prerequisite to satisfactory manipulation of the joint. In many cases injury occurs when the legs become anchored due to studs in the boots. If rotation of the trunk is superimposed onto this static lower limb situation the stress imposed on the knee joint is enormous. The application of NMT prior to attempting correction not only makes the correction less painful but ensures that the result is lasting. NMT is also beneficial in the treatment of prepatellar bursitis, and any synovial inflammatory problems.

A problem which plagues many sportsmen, particularly footballers, basketball players and volleyball players, is pain in the groin and down the inside of the leg. This is commonly treated as a sacroiliac or a lumbar problem when, in many cases, it is due to a lesion of the symphysis-pubis. There are a number of techniques for dealing with problems of this joint but none so dramatically successful as the application of NMT.

The technique's effectiveness in producing long-term benefits is perhaps best underlined by the results with sportsmen such as Roger Uttley and Gerry Francis, who had both received short-term benefit from manipulative treatment. The application of NMT, without any change in the manipulative techniques being employed, except to make them less specific, produced long-term improvement which allowed a return to active participation in their respective sports. In both cases the main problem was an imbalance in muscle tone with excessive tension causing persistence of the joint dysfunction. The removal of these soft tissue factors restored balance and encouraged the body to return to normal function, as it always tries to do.

In summary, the benefits of NMT in general are (1) that it is a technique which removes causes rather than dealing with symptoms. (2) It removes the necessity for the bulk of specific manipulation, instead it encourages the body to normalize itself. (3) It is applicable to any part of the body. From the specific sports injury point of view the main advantage of NMT is that it provides (1) a more rapid recovery rate and (2) a more permanent one.

My own experience confirms the validity of Terry Moule's comments. NMT apart from all the myriad applications discussed in earlier chapters, is the finest soft tissue system for helping to normalize acute and chronic injuries. In the past 20 years I have used these methods on tens of thousands of patients. In many cases sporting and theatrical performers have been restored to normal in a short space of time. Where the 'show must go on'—and in present terms this applies to athletic and sporting performance just as much as to theatrical performance—time is vital. NMT and the various methods that may accompany it, such as ultrasonics, manipulation, hydrotherapy, exercise, cryotherapy etc. have been successful time after time. I have found NMT invaluable in dealing with acute injuries affecting such personalities as Richard Burton (acute torticollis during the filming of *Look Back in Anger*), James Booth (acute low back during the West End run of *Fings Ai'nt What They Used To Be*), Christopher Neame (neck injury sustained in fall from balcony during *Romeo and Juliet*), Bryan Forbes (neck strain during filming of *League of Gentlemen*), Harry Andrews (fell off horse during filming of *Devil's Disciple*).

All of these were able to resume work within one day of the injury. In all cases no proper treatment facilities were available. Conditions ranged from the dressing room floor for James Booth to the lush grass of Tring Park for Harry Andrews. No equipment was available other than my hands and no treatment was used other than NMT and gentle mobilization. The economy, versatility and effectiveness of NMT has proved itself over and over again. In more chronic conditions NMT has proved equally useful on countless occasions.

The successful use of NMT calls for the applied thought of the practitioner. The body responds rapidly to the help this technique offers. Its limitations are almost always related to the limitations of the practitioner. Its success is in direct proportion to the dedication and intelligence with which it is applied.

Bibliography

Barlow, W., 'Anxiety and Muscle Tension Pain,' *British Journal of Clinical Practice,* Vol. 3, No. 5.

Becker, Alan R., 'Parameters of Resistance', *Journal of the American Osteopathic Association* (Sept. 1973), p. 39.

Blashy, M., 'Manipulation of the Neuromuscular Unit via the Periphery of the CNS', *Southern Medical Journal* (Aug. 1961).

Boadella, David, 'The Language of the Body in Bio-energetic Therapy', *Journal of the Research Society for Natural Therapeutics* (1978).

Cathie, Dr A., 'Selected Writings,' *Academy of Applied Osteopathy Yearbook* (1974).

Chaitow, Leon, 'An Introduction to Chapman's Reflexes', *British Naturopathic Journal* (Spring 1965).

——*The Acupuncture Treatment of Pain* (Thorsons Publishers Limited, Wellingborough, Northants, 1976).

Cooper, Gerald J., 'Considerations on Fascia in Diagnosis and Treatment', *Journ. of Amer. Ost. Assoc.,* Vol. 78 (Jan. 1979), pp. 336-73.

Cyriax, J., *Textbook of Orthopaedic Medicine,* Vols 1 and 2 (Balliere).

Dittrich, R. J., 'Somatic Pain and Autonomic Concomitants', *American Journal of Surgery* (1954).

Ebner, M., *Connective Tissue Massage* (Churchill Livingstone, 1962).*

Erlinghauser, R. F., 'Circulation of CSF through Connective Tissue', *Academy of Applied Osteopathy Yearbook* (1959).

Fielder and Pyott, *The Science and Art of Manipulative Surgery* (American Institute of Manipulative Surgery Inc., 1955).

Gustein, R., 'The Role of Abdominal Fibrositis in Functional Indigestion', *Mississippi Valley Medical Journal,* 66 (1944), p. 114.

—— A Review of Myodysneuria (Fibrositis)', *American Practitioner and Digest of Treatments,* Vol. 6, No. 4.

——'The Role Craniocervical Myodysneuria in Functional Ocular Disorders', *American Practitioner and Digest of Treatments* (Nov. 1956).

Hagbarth, K., 'Excitatory and Inhibitory Skin Areas for Flexor and Extensor Motoneurons', *Acta Physiologia Scandinavia* (1952).

*Now available in a revised edition from Krieger Publishing Co., Inc., U.S.A.

Jacobson, E., 'Principles Underlying Coronary Heart Disease', *Cardiologia* (1956), pp. 16-83.

Jones, L. H., 'Foot Treatment Without Hand Trauma', *Journ. Amer. Ost. Assoc.* (July, 1963).

Korr, I., 'Spinal Cord as Organiser of Disease Process', *Academy of Applied Osteopathy Yearbook* (1976).

Lawson-Wood, D. and Lawson-Wood, J., *Progressive Vitality and Dynamic Posture* (Health Science Press, 1978).

Little, K. E., 'Toward More Effective Manipulative Management of Chronic Myofascial Strain and Stress Syndromes', *Journal of the Academy of Applied Osteopathy,* Vol. 68 (March, 1969).

Mennel, J., 'The Therapeutic Use of Cold', *Journ. Amer. Ost. Assoc.,* Vol. 74 (Aug. 1975).

Patterson, M., 'Model Mechanism for Spinal Segmental Facilitation', *Academy of Applied Osteopathy Yearbook* (1976).

Reich, Wilhelm, *Character Analysis* (Vision Press).

Rolf, Ida, 'Structural Dynamics', *Academy of Applied Osteopathy Yearbook* (1962).

Selye, H., *The Stress of Life* (McGraw Hill, 1956).

Stoddard, A., *Manual of Osteopathic Practice* (Hutchinson, 1969).

Taylor, R. B., 'Bioenergetics of Man', *Academy of Applied Osteopathy Yearbook* (1958).

Travell, J., 'Ethyl Chloride Spray for Painful Muscle Spasm', *Arch. Phys. Med. Rehabl.,* 33 (May, 1952), pp. 291-8.

——'Symposium on Mechanism and Management of Pain Syndromes', *Proc. Rudolph Virchow Medical Society* (1957).

Travell, J., and Bigelow, N., 'Role of Somatic Trigger Areas in Patterns of Hysteria', *Psychosomatic Medicine,* Vol. 9, No. 6.

Webber, T. D., 'Diagnosis and Modification of Headache and Shoulder, Arm, Hand Syndromes', *Journ. Amer. Ost. Assoc.,* Vol. 72 (March, 1973).

Youngs, B., 'NMT of Lower Thorax and Low Back', *British Naturopathic Journal,* Vol. 5, No. 11.

——'Physiological Background of N.M. Technique', *British Naturopathic Journal,* Vol. 5, No. 6.

Index